# Comprehensive Diabetes Care

## Awareness, Prevention, and Treatment

snova
New York

# Endocrinology Research and Clinical Developments Series

**Receptor-Targeted Therapies in Diabetes Mellitus: From Pathophysiology to Innovative Treatments**
Ajmer Singh Grewal, PhD,
Neelam Singh, PhD,
Swati Verma,
Chaitanay Vinayak Narayan,
and Ashutosh Kumar Verma
ISBN: 979-8-89530-587-4
eBook ISBN: 979-8-89530-653-6

**Naturally Occurring Chemicals for the Treatment and Management of Diabetes Mellitus and Related Disorders**
Ajmer Singh Grewal, PhD,
Geeta Deswal, PhD,
Ashwani K. Dhingra, PhD,
Priyanka Kriplani, PhD,
Bhawna Chopra, PhD,
and Shikha Baghel Chauhan, PhD
ISBN: 979-8-89113-491-1
eBook ISBN: 979-8-89113-613-7

**Diabetes: Research, Economic Impact, and New Programs**
Lisa Primitiva (Editor)
ISBN: 979-8-89113-545-1
eBook ISBN: 979-8-89113-620-5

**Management of Diabetes Mellitus Based on Natural Products**
Yachana Mishra, PhD,
and Vijay Mishra, PhD
ISBN: 979-8-88697-853-7
eBook ISBN: 979-8-88697-970-1

**The Biochemical Guide to Hormones**
David Aebisher, PhD, DSc
ISBN: 979-8-88697-492-8
eBook ISBN: 979-8-88697-534-5

**Understanding and Managing Hyperthyroidism**
Poongkodi Karunakaran, PhD
ISBN: 979-8-88697-636-6
eBook ISBN: 979-8-88697-648-9

**More information about this series can be found at**
https://novapublishers.com/product-category/series/endocrinology-research-and-clinical-developments/

**Joseph S. Green**
Editor

# Comprehensive Diabetes Care

## Awareness, Prevention, and Treatment

snova
New York

**Library of Congress Cataloging-in-Publication Data**

ISBN: 979-8-89530-772-4 (Hardcover)
ISBN: 979-8-89530-948-3 (eBook)

*Published by Nova Science Publishers, Inc. † New York*

# Contents

# Preface

Diabetes affects over 37 million Americans—about one in ten—and an additional 96 million adults live with prediabetes. With rates steadily rising, an alarming one in three Americans is projected to develop diabetes in their lifetime. Beyond being a serious condition on its own, diabetes significantly contributes to heart disease, stroke, amputations, blindness, and kidney failure—carving out an enormous impact on individuals and society alike. Yet, the power to change this trajectory lies in prevention and management. By taking informed steps, you can reduce your risk and lead a healthier, more empowered life.

# Chapter 1

# What Is Fueling the Diabetes Epidemic?*

## Committee on Health, Education, Labor, and Pensions

Thursday, December 14, 2023

U.S. Senate, Committee on Health, Education, Labor, and Pensions,
*Washington, DC.*

The Committee met, pursuant to notice, at 10:02 a.m., in room 430, Dirksen Senate Office Building, Hon. Bernard Sanders, Chairman of the Committee, presiding.

Present: Senators Sanders [presiding], Casey, Baldwin, Kaine, Hassan, Smith, Hickenlooper, Cassidy, Collins, Braun, Marshall, and Budd.

## Opening Statement of Senator Sanders

The CHAIR. Senate Committee on Health, Education, Labor, and Pensions will come to order. Today, we are going to be discussing one of the major health crises in America, and that is the diabetes epidemic that is having a huge impact on our Country and an issue that must be addressed.

Diabetes, as I think we all know, is not only a serious illness unto itself, but it is a contributing factor to heart disease, stroke, amputations, blindness, and

* This is an edited, reformatted and augmented version of Hearing of the Committee on Health, Education, Labor, and Pensions United States Senate, One Hundred Eighteenth Congress First Session on Examining the Diabetes Epidemic, Publication No. S. HRG. 118–211, dated December 14, 2023.

In: Comprehensive Diabetes Care
Editor: Joseph S. Green
ISBN: 979-8-89530-772-4

kidney failure. Type 1 diabetes is a major problem that impacts over 1.4 million Americans, and we are going to be discussing that issue today.

My understanding is that Senator Cassidy has brought two witnesses who are extremely knowledgeable about type 1 diabetes, and we look forward to hearing what they have to say. My focus is going to be on type 2 diabetes, which impacts about 95 percent of Americans who have diabetes.

There is obviously a whole lot that can be said about diabetes, but here are just a few of the questions that I hope we will dive into this morning. First, and maybe most importantly, why have we seen a huge increase in the number of people in America who have developed diabetes over the last 50 years? What is going on? What has changed?

I think that may be the most important question. Second, how is diabetes impacting our healthcare system? And I think we know some of those answers. Thirdly, given the huge number of people who are struggling with diabetes, how can we make the treatments, and there are some very effective treatments out there how do we make them available to everyone who needs them regardless of their income?

Further, when we talk about the cost of treatments and diabetes, we are cognizant of the fact that Medicaid and Medicare and other public health programs spend huge amounts of money for those treatments, as do private health insurance companies. So how do we make sure that we don't bankrupt Medicare and Medicaid in the process of treating diabetes? First, the problem.

Today in America, rather remarkably, we have over 35 million Americans, that is over 10 percent of our population, who have type 2 diabetes. And the cost of treating that disease is absolutely staggering. According to the American Diabetes Association, the total cost of diabetes in the United States was nearly $413 billion last year, $413 billion, and that is up 27 percent over the past 6 years.

That amounts to about 10 percent of our overall health care costs. So, $1 out of every $10 spent on health care is dealing with diabetes. And when we talk about the type 2 diabetes epidemic and the huge increase in new cases, we must also talk about another epidemic, and that is the epidemic of obesity in America.

Some 90 percent of people with type 2 diabetes are overweight or obese. These two epidemics go hand in hand. A key question that we must discuss. How did it happen, according to the CDC, that the rate of childhood obesity in America has tripled since the 1970's, tripled since the 1970's, and has gotten so bad that one out of every five children, and over 40 percent of adults in our Country, today are now obese?

Why is it that, according to the CDC, the number of children in America with type 2 diabetes is estimated to skyrocket by nearly 700 percent over the next 40 years unless we get a handle on that issue. Isn't that just an extraordinary number?

The answers to those questions are not complicated. Difficult, but not complicated.

For decades, in my view, we have allowed large corporations in the food and beverage industry to entice children to eat foods and beverages loaded up with sugar, salt, and saturated fat purposely designed to be overeaten. The situation has gotten so bad that most of what children in America eat today consist of unhealthy, ultra processed foods that doctors have told us lead to a higher risk of type 2 diabetes.

Alarmingly, according to a recent study that will be discussed this morning, ultra-processed foods, which make up an incredible 73 percent of our Nation's food supply, can be as addicted—addictive, can be as addictive as alcohol and nearly as addictive as cigarettes.

While diabetes and obesity rates in America soar, while we spend hundreds of billions of dollars to treat diabetes, the food and beverage industry spent $14 billion last year on advertising to make many of their unhealthy products appealing to the American consumer.

Even worse, and I think really what gets to me, $2 billion of their advertising budget is used to directly market food predominantly high in sugar, salt, and saturated fat to our children in order to get them hooked on these products at an early age.

How is that? According to the Rudd Center for Food Policy and Obesity, children and teens view about 4,000 food and beverage ads on television every year, an average of 10 advertisements each day. Another study found that children who watch Nickelodeon and Nicktoons are exposed to over 10 unhealthy food and beverage ads every hour, they're going after the children. Let me give you just one example.

Last year, for example, Coca Cola spent $327 million on advertising in the United States alone. Not one of those ads will tell you that drinking one or two cans of Coke a day will increase your chances of getting type 2 diabetes by 26 percent. I didn't quite see that in those lovely ads that they do.

Nor will their TV ads tell you that one 20 ounce bottle of Coke contains over 15 teaspoons of sugar, more than twice the recommended daily limit for kids under the age of 18. Nearly 30 years ago, as I think we all know and the American people know, Congress had the extraordinary courage and it was not easy to take on the tobacco industry, whose products killed over 400,000 Americans every year, including my father.

Congress had the courage to do that then. Now is the time for us to seriously combat the type 2 diabetes and obesity epidemics in America. In order to do that, we must have the courage to take on the greed of the food and beverage industry, which every day is undermining the health and well-being of our children.

As adults, as responsible people, as representatives of the American people, we have got to do that. And in my view, a good place to start would be to ban junk food ads targeted to children. Now, this is not a radical idea.

The NIH has estimated that if the United States banned fast food advertising marketed to children, talking about kids, we could cut the childhood obesity rate in our Country by up to 18 percent.

In the 1980's, Quebec banned junk food advertising to children. Today, Quebec has the lowest childhood obesity rate in Canada and the highest consumption of fruits and vegetables of any province in their nation.

Ireland, Sweden, South Korea, Taiwan, Spain, Portugal, and several other major countries throughout the world have either seriously restricted or banned junk food ads targeted to children.

In addition to addressing the causes of type 2 diabetes, there is another important issue that we have got to address. We have got to make certain that the treatments available to people with diabetes are affordable for all Americans and are not bankrupting Federal health insurance programs or raising the cost of private insurance.

The very good news is that a new class of treatments for diabetes and obesity like Ozempic and Mounjaro have the potential to be a game changer with respect to these major epidemics. According to clinical trials, these drugs, which suppress appetite, have been estimated to help people lose 15 to 20 percent of their weight.

That is the good news, and it is importantly good news. The bad news is that these drugs also have the potential to bankrupt Medicare and the American people. According to research published in the New England Journal of Medicine, if just 10 percent of people with obesity on Medicare took these drugs, it could cost Medicare up to $27 billion a year, driving Medicare premiums way, way up.

Further, incredibly, these drugs, Ozempic and Mounjaro are up to 15 times more expensive in the United States than they are in other major countries. Let me repeat, these two important drugs, up to 15 times more expensive in the United States than in other countries. Ozempic, manufactured by Novo Nordisk, cost $12,000 a year in the United States. Do you know what it costs in Germany? $750 a year.

Mounjaro, manufactured by Eli Lilly, costs $13,000 in the United States, costs $2,000 a year in the United Kingdom. Incredibly, it has been estimated that Eli Lilly, Novo Nordisk, and others in the pharmaceutical industry stand to make as much as $150 billion off of these drugs each and every year by charging us by far the highest prices in the world for their products.

This is, to my mind, unacceptable for so many reasons, and that is why I am going to be introducing legislation which is very simple. It is legislation that says that here in the United States, we cannot continue to pay the highest prices in the world for prescription drugs. We should not be paying more than other major countries.

If that bill were to be signed into law, we would lower the cost of prescription drugs in this country by 50 percent. So, that is where we are today. We have two issues. What is the cause of the epidemic, and how do we make sure that we have treatments available to all?

I very much thank all of the panelists for being here. This is a very important issue and I look forward to this discussion.

Senator Cassidy, the mic is yours.

## Opening Statement of Senator Cassidy

Senator CASSIDY. Thank you, Chairman Sanders. The obesity epidemic is quite remarkable. And type 1 diabetes obviously not related to obesity, but nonetheless, part of that which we are addressing today.

If you look at a kind of a map of the United States over the last three decades and the prevalence and incidence of diabetes, it just lights up. Goes bigger and more intense, etcetera, however you look at the map. So, it is a bipartisan issue. I am glad the Committee is addressing it.

I will say, however, that the focus of the hearing has changed from our original agreement to explore the prevention, treatment, and management of diabetes from a clinical and public health perspective.

Diet and access to healthy foods are important, but I will point out that corporate marketing practices to consumers and human nutrition are not the jurisdiction of this Committee. Those are on the Commerce and Agriculture.

Food marketing is what this Committee will focus on today, but ideally, the Committee's time would be addressing issues over which we have legislative authority. If we have legislative authority, we can do something. If we have a hearing on something over which we have no legislative authority, we have a hearing.

I will also point out, though, that our colleagues, Senator Susan Collins and Jeanne Shaheen have led the Special Diabetes Program Reauthorization, which the Committee did successfully vote out in June. When enacted, it will provide additional mandatory resources for diabetes research at NIH.

I would also like, and that would be a good thing to have discuss today, how the NIH is using its discretionary funding, because that is something over which we do actually have jurisdiction. We should look at why NIH habitually under funds obesity research, despite it being the kind of foundation of why the rate of type 2 diabetes has gone up so dramatically, as well as, by the way, its impact upon many other medical conditions.

It is important to explore the impact of recent medical advances upon the lives of diabetics. American medical innovation is saving countless lives. Diabetes is no different. Groundbreaking developments in diabetes management like the continuous glucose monitor, or CGM, increases patient adherence to treatment while improving quality of life for patients and peace of mind for parents and caretakers.

We could familiarize ourselves more with that. I am a doc, but I wasn't aware of it. And then somebody says, oh, you look on your phone and you see what your diabetes is. It kind of really brings it home to the folks.

It was quite remarkable. My internist friends explaining to me how this has been so positive of a change in terms of the management of diabetes. We can point out that even 10 years ago, parents were worried about their children developing diabetic shock.

But now, with affordable CGMs and other innovative devices, blood glucose levels are monitored in real time, and these devastating occurrences, such as diabetic shock, are prevented.

We need to continue to foster innovation and the solutions it creates. CGM are miracles to many now, but at some point it will become yesterday's news. We need the next miracles. Cellular treatments are on the horizon, and we have the potential to again revolutionize how Americans live with diabetes.

I visited an outfit in Massachusetts, and they showed me this kind of twirling bath, and they said those are islet cells that can be gathered up and injected under someone's arm, and this is a technology that will be implemented. Quite remarkable. Again, we could have been discussing that today.

The task of this Committee is to balance affordability with innovation. I accept the Chair's point. If there is an innovation that someone cannot afford, it is as if that innovation doesn't occur.

I am with you on that. But we should again be discussing topics within the Committee's jurisdiction. That is what we have the responsibility to do. And if there is something that we can actually address, then consider legislation.

I look forward to exploring the issues that we can address with our witnesses. With that, I yield.

The CHAIR. Thank you very much, Senator Cassidy. Now we are going to hear from our very distinguished and knowledgeable witnesses, and we are delighted they are with us today. Our first witness will be Dr. Ashley Gearhardt, who is a Professor of Psychology and Clinical Science at the University of Michigan.

Dr. Gearhardt's research focuses on the effects of poor nutrition on diabetes and obesity, and factors driving excessive consumption of unhealthy foods. Notably, she has published a recent study on how ultra-processed foods can be as addictive as nicotine and alcohol. Dr. Gearhardt, thanks so much for being with us.

## Statement of Ashley Gearhardt, PhD, Professor of Psychology, University of Michigan, Ann Arbor, MI

Dr. GEARHARDT. Chairman Sanders, Ranking Member Cassidy, and distinguished Members of the Committee, thank you for the opportunity to participate in today's meeting.

To begin, I will briefly review my qualifications to speak as an expert at this hearing. I received my Ph.D. in Clinical Psychology at Yale University with a focus on addictive disorders, obesity, and disordered eating.

I am currently a Professor of Psychology and the Director of the Food and Addiction Science and Treatment Lab at the University of Michigan. I am also a licensed clinical psychologist. Through my clinical experiences, I have gained a firsthand understanding of how hard people are working to try and get control over their eating.

I saw that even when people were faced with life threatening health conditions like diabetes and were very motivated to change, they still failed to do so. My research has been built on the parallels between what I observed in the clinic and my scientific training on how certain substances can trigger addictive processes.

In my research I use multi-method approaches to explore the neuro-biological, psychological, and behavioral factors that contribute to compulsive overeating and its negative consequences like obesity and diabetes. The American food supply has changed dramatically over the last 40 years.

The American diet is now composed mostly of ultra-processed foods. Ultra-processed foods are industrially manufactured products created by deconstructing foods from their component parts, modifying them, and combining them with a myriad of additives.

The resulting ultra-processed foods contain little, if any, whole foods, and they are a major source of added sugars and saturated fats in our diets. The average American adult and child gets the majority of their calories from ultra-processed foods.

Ultra-processed foods have been implicated in health conditions like depression and obesity across numerous studies. Based on analysis of 400,000 people, every 10 percent increase in ultra-processed food intake is associated with a 12 percent higher risk of type 2 diabetes.

There are strong parallels between addictive substances and ultra-processed foods. Addictive substances are created through processing natural substances like fruits or leaves into new prod ucts that rapidly deliver a naturally high doses of reinforcing ingredients into the body like nicotine and cigarettes.

Ultra-processed foods are similarly created by altering natural substances like fruits and grains into products that deliver a naturally high doses and combinations of carbohydrates and fats, which are then rapidly digested by our bodies.

Additives further enhance the flavor and texture of these ultraprocessed foods and make them shelf stable, accessible, and convenient. Basic neuroscience finds that ultra-processed foods high in carbohydrates and fats activate reward systems in the brain in an analogous manner to addictive substances like nicotine.

Key signs of addiction occur in our intake of ultra-processed foods. Systematic reviews of over 280 studies estimate that 14 percent of adults and 12 percent of children meet the criteria for an addictive disorder in their intake of ultra-processed foods.

This includes losing control over intake, intense, almost irresistible cravings, and an inability to reduce intake despite serious negative consequences. This addictive pattern of ultra-processed food intake is associated with a more than five times greater occurrence of type 2 diabetes. I want to provide a representative quote from a research participant from my lab.

She said, I can't even be in the same vicinity as a donut store or any type of donuts because I will finish a dozen all by myself, and I am a type 2 diabetic so that could kill me. I know that, and I know that I shouldn't be eating all of those. I shouldn't be eating one, let alone a whole dozen, but for some reason I just can't stop eating them.

If addictive mechanisms are being triggered by ultra-processed foods, this may be an overlooked reason why it can be challenging to reduce intake even in the face of health conditions like diabetes. There are also strong connections between the tobacco and processed food industries.

From the 1980's to the late 2000, tobacco companies like R.J. Reynolds and Philip Morris became the biggest producers of processed food in the world. Internal tobacco industry documents demonstrate strategies designed to develop and sell cigarettes were applied to their processed food and beverage holdings, such as adding flavor enhancers developed for cigarettes into children's sugar sweetened beverages and increasing targeted marketing to children and racial ethnic minorities.

Lessons learned from the tobacco epidemic can help guide solutions here. Investing in science to understand how ultra-processed foods activate mechanisms of addiction and contribute to excessive intake is important.

Multi-pronged approaches and a focus on prevention, particularly for youth, will be important for improving Americans' health. Thank you for your time.

[The prepared statement of Dr. Gearhardt follows:]

## Prepared Statement of Ashley Gearhardt

### Introduction

Chairman Sanders, Ranking Member Cassidy, and Distinguished Members of the Committee: thank you for the opportunity to participate in today's hearing. To begin, I will briefly review my qualifications to speak as an expert at today's hearing. I received my PhD in clinical psychology at Yale University with a focus on addictive disorders, obesity, and disordered eating. I have spent 11 years on the faculty at the University of Michigan. I am currently a professor of psychology and the director of the Food and Addiction Science Treatment laboratory at that institution. I am also a licensed clinical psychologist who has provided treatment to individuals with substance use disorders, obesity, and compulsive overeating.

Through my clinical experiences, I have gained a firsthand understanding of how hard people are working to try and get control over their eating behavior. I saw that even when people were faced with life threatening health conditions, they often still failed to reduce their intake of highly palatable foods despite being motivated to change. My research has been built on the parallels between what I observed in the clinic and my scientific training on how certain substances can trigger addictive processes that keep people stuck in compulsive and destructive patterns of consumption. In my program of research, I use multi-method approaches to explore the neurobiological, psychological, and behavioral factors that contribute to compulsive overeating across the lifespan. I have published over 175 peer-reviewed articles, including in prestigious outlets like the JAMA Psychiatry and British Medical Journal.

### Ultra-Processed Foods Dominate the American Diet

The modern American diet is now composed mostly of ultra-processed foods [1, 2], which are industrial formulations manufactured by deconstructing foods into their component parts, modifying them and recombining them with a myriad of additives [3–5]. Common examples of ultra-processed foods are industrially created candy, sugar-sweetened carbonated beverages, instant noodles, frozen pizza, and salty snacks [4]. Ultra-processed foods are a distinct category from minimally processed foods (e.g., fruit, vegetables) that have been washed, chopped, frozen, dried or fermented and processed culinary ingredients used for home cooking (e.g., butter, flour).

Ultra-processed foods are a major source of added sugar and saturated fats in the American diet [6, 7]. Most ultra-processed foods are considered hyperalatable due to their unnaturally high level of palatability-inducing nutrients (fats, sugars, carbohydrates and/or sodium), which trigger reward signals and reduce sensitivity to satiety signals [1, 8]. Ultra-processed foods also often contain flavor additives and texturizers that enhance taste and the feel of the product in the mouth [3–5]. The preservatives in many ultra-processed foods allow them to stay shelf-stable and come in convenient ready-to-heat or ready-to-eat packages [3–5]. Epidemiological research estimates that the average American adult now gets the majority of their calories (57 percent) from ultra-processed foods while intake of nutrient-rich minimally processed foods like fruits, vegetables, and legumes is decreasing [2]. This estimate is even higher for youth. From 1999 to 2018, a global team of epidemiologists found that the percentage of energy consumed from ultra-processed foods increased from 61.4 percent to 67.0 percent in children 2 to 19 years old [9].

A converging body of research highlights the potential ramifications of diets composed of high levels of ultra-processed foods [10]. High levels of ultra-processed food intake have been implicated in an increased prevalence of health conditions like depression, heart disease, and obesity [10]. In a controlled randomized crossover trial, a team of researchers at the National Institute of Health found that being given a diet high in ultra-processed foods relative to minimally processed foods over a 2- week period was associated with an increased daily intake of 500 calories and a two-pound weight gain [11]. This occurred despite the ultra-processed and minimally processed meals being matched on the overall calories available to participants [11]. Furthermore, a meta-analysis of over 400,000 participants found that every 10 percent increase in ultra-processed food intake was associated with a 12 percent higher risk of Type 2 diabetes [12]. Thus, the high levels of ultra-processed food in the American diet are a major cause for concern and may be contributing to the obesity and diabetes epidemics.

## There are Strong Parallels between Addictive Substances and Ultra-Processed Foods

Most addictive substances are created by processing natural substances (e.g., fruit, leaves) into a new product that delivers a heighted dose of a reinforcing ingredient (e.g., ethanol, nicotine) into the body [13]. Speed of absorption is also important and the more rapidly the reinforcing ingredient is absorbed the more likely the substance is to be addictive [14, 15]. All addictive substances activate the mesolimbic dopamine system, which is key to the reward and motivational mechanisms that go awry in addiction [16, 17]. For example, cigarettes are created by processing naturally occurring tobacco leaves through drying and curing into products that can be smoked to rapidly deliver high doses of nicotine into the body. The nicotine in cigarettes is further amplified by flavor enhancers, such as sugar, cocoa, and menthol, which create brand-specific taste and flavor profiles [18, 19]. These tastes and flavors become repeatedly paired with the delivery of nicotine and become salient drivers of smoking behavior in their own right [18, 19]. The cigarettes that result from this processing are highly addictive and can lead people to continue smoking even when facing life-threatening health conditions, like heart disease and lung cancer [20].

Similarly, many ultra-processed foods are created by processing naturally occurring substances (e.g., fruits, grains, vegetables) into products that deliver unnaturally high doses of rapidly absorbed carbohydrates and/or fats. Refined carbohydrates, like sugar, and fat are highly reinforcing ingredients and they are effective at activating reward mechanisms in the brain [13, 21–23]. While many minimally processed foods contain either carbohydrate (e.g., fruit) or fat (e.g., nuts, meat), the combination of both is rare in nature [21]. In contrast, ultra-processed foods often deliver high levels of both refined carbohydrates and fats. This combination has a supra-additive effect in activating neural reward systems [22]. Evidence exists that sugar, fat, and ultra-processed foods can activate mesolimbic dopamine in the brain at similar magnitudes as nicotine and ethanol [24–29]. Additives further amplify ultra-processed foods by coupling industry created flavors and textures with the delivery of refined carbohydrates and added fats [4, 5]. Thus, these ultraprocessed foods with high levels of refined carbohydrates and fats are highly rewarding processed substances that share many commonalities with addictive substances like cigarettes [13].

## Ultra-Processed Food Addiction

A common set of diagnostic criteria are used to identify individuals who are experiencing clinically significant problems with addictive substances (see Table 1), including a loss of control over intake, intense cravings, and continue consumption despite physical or emotional problems [30]. In 2008, my colleagues and I developed the Yale Food Addiction Scale, which applies these same criteria to the intake of ultra-processed foods (e.g., chocolate, soda, French fries, pizza) [31]. The Yale Food Addiction Scale has been extensively validated and is a widely used measure in the field with over 1000 citations and translations available in over a dozen languages [32]. When we first began this research, the concept of ultra-processed foods was just emerging and investigations into what types of foods were consumed addictively was limited. Given the dearth of research at that time, we used the term ''food addiction'' to reflect meeting the diagnostic criteria for a substance use disorder in the realm of food intake. Since that time, it has become clear that not all foods are consumed addictively. Multiple studies have identified that people report consuming ultra-processed foods high in refined carbohydrates and/or fats in an addictive manner, but not minimally processed foods like fruits, vegetables, and legumes [33–35]. Dietary intake studies confirm that individuals who meet ''food addiction'' consume higher levels of ultra-processed foods, but lower levels of minimally processed foods [36, 37]. Thus, I will refer to the construct measured by the Yale Food Addiction Scale as ultra-processed food addiction in the remainder of my testimony.

Although ultra-processed food addiction is not currently an officially recognized diagnosis by the American Psychiatric Association, the science on this topic has grown quickly. Systematic reviews of over 280 studies from 36 different countries estimate the prevalence of ultra-processed food addiction to be 14 percent in adults [38], which is similar to the prevalence of alcohol and tobacco use disorder (e.g., 14 percent for alcohol and 18 percent for tobacco) [39, 40]. The estimated prevalence of ultra-processed food addiction is twice as high (28 percent) in adults with obesity (38). Particularly relevant to the current hearing, ultra-processed food addiction has been associated with a more than five times greater likelihood of Type 2 diabetes even when adjusting for sex and age [41].

Below is a quote from a participant who was interviewed for a research study in my lab about their experience with ultra-processed food addiction.

''I can't even be in the same vicinity as [donut store] or any type of donuts, 'cause I will finish a dozen all by myself and I'm type 2 diabetic. So, that could kill me, and I know that and I know that I shouldn't be eating all those. I shouldn't be eating one, let alone a whole dozen. But for some reason I just can't stop eating them.''

In children, the estimated prevalence for ultra-processed food addiction based on a systematic review of the literature is 12 percent, which surpasses the prevalence of other substance addictions at this stage of development [42]. Children are typically protected against exposure to addictive substances through policy initiatives (e.g., marketing restrictions, age limits on purchases), but exposure to ultra-processed foods for children in America is a daily occurrence [9]. There is also evidence that ultra-processed food addiction is important for older Americans. In collaboration with Michigan Medicine, my lab recently conducted a study on ultra-processed food addiction in the National Poll of Healthy Aging. This is a nationally representative poll of over 2000 older adults between the ages of 50 and 80. In this poll, 13 percent of participants met the criteria for a clinically significant ultra-processed food addiction, which was associated with a greater likelihood of reporting being overweight and in poorer physical and mental health [43]. Finally, individuals with food insecurity that lack adequate access to nutritious food are more than three times more likely to meet the criteria for ultra-processed food addiction with chips, soda, chocolate, pizza, and ice cream being identified as the most addictive foods [35].

Taken together, this scientific body of evidence suggests that addictive processes play an important role in contributing to patterns of ultra-processed food intake implicated in poor health obesity, and diabetes [21, 44]. If addictive mechanisms are being triggered by ultra-processed foods, this may be an overlooked reason why it can be challenging to reduce intake of ultra-processed foods even in the face of health conditions like diabetes.

## Connections between the Tobacco and Processed Food/Beverage Industries

The industries that profit from tobacco and ultra-processed foods are interconnected. In the 1970's and 1980's, the tobacco companies RJ Reynolds and Philip Morris bought processed food and beverage companies, including Kraft and General Foods [45, 46]. When Philip Morris merged Kraft and General Foods in 1987, it became the largest processed food corporation in the world [45, 46]. Although the tobacco industry sold off many of their holdings in this arena by the late 2000's [45, 46], they had already impacted the nature of the

American food supply. Internal tobacco industry documents demonstrate they took strategies designed to develop and sell cigarettes and applied them to their processed food and beverage products [45, 46]. This includes putting flavor additives developed to enhance the palatability of cigarettes in their leading children's sugar-sweetened drinks and increasing marketing strategies that targeted children and racial/ethnic minorities [45, 46]. A recent study published in the journal Addiction found that between 1988 to 2001 products from tobacco-owned food companies were significantly more likely to have foods with hyper-palatable combinations of carbohydrates, fat, and salt compared to foods from non-tobacco owned companies [47]. However, by 2018, non-tobacco owned food companies had increased their level of hyper-palatable foods to levels that compared with tobacco-owned companies [47]. This contributed to a modern food supply composed largely of ultra-processed, hyper-palatable foods [1]. During this same time period, the amount of diabetes doubled (48) and the presence of moderate-to-high risk obesity tripled in America [49].

## What Can Be Done to Address this Problem?

Tobacco also provides a point of reference on how we might reduce the costs associated with excessive intake of ultra-processed foods. Even when the health consequences of smoking became more evident, it took decades for their addictive nature to be acknowledged. Tobacco can look different than other addictive substances, as it does not induce a clear intoxication syndrome and is legal and accessible. In part, because of these differences, the addictive nature of tobacco products was hotly debated for decades despite thousands of tobacco-related deaths occurring each year [20, 50]. Eventually, consensus was reached that tobacco products were addictive based in large part on scientific evidence on their highly reinforcing nature and their ability to trigger compulsive patterns of use [20]. A similar debate now exists about the addictive nature of ultra-processed foods [13].

Cigarettes are complex substances with up to 4000 different chemicals and even now the exact dose at which nicotine can trigger addiction in unknown [13]. However, research has investigated how different aspects of cigarettes interact to increase their addictiveness. In addition to the dose of nicotine, additives and delivery mechanisms that speed up the absorption of nicotine appear to increase the addictiveness of cigarettes [18, 19, 51]. Processes that enhance the taste and flavor of tobacco products (e.g., sugar, menthol, cocoa) have also been identified as important contributors to their addictive nature [18, 19]. Investing in similar research to unpack how different aspects of ultra-processed foods interact to activate mechanisms of addiction and contribute to excessive patterns of intake will be important. This science could provide guidance to inform consumers about the risks associated with different types of ultra-processed foods and could guide targets for different policy approaches.

A wide range of potential approaches are available for consideration to reduce excessive intake of ultra-processed foods to improve the health of Americans. The history of addressing addiction epidemics also suggest that no singular approach will be sufficient to address complex public health like the obesity and diabetes epidemic. However, multi-pronged strategies have been effective in reducing the costs associated with addictive substances. In the context of tobacco, combining approaches like educational programs, labeling, economic incentives, age restrictions and marketing limitations helped drastically lower smoking rates in America [52– 54]. Countries, such as Chile and the United Kingdom, are instituting similar approaches to address the epidemic of diet-related disease, such as limiting marketing for less healthy foods to children. It is also not just people who experience clinically impairing levels of ultra-processed food addiction who would likely benefit. When addictive substances are inexpensive, easily accessible, and heavily marketed, many people without a clinical level of addiction are still prone to consume these substances excessively and experience problems in their mental or physical health. Thus, widespread use of addictive substances that stay below the clinical threshold for diagnosis can still pose a significant public health burden [55]. On average, Americans experience between one to two symptoms of addiction in their intake of ultra-processed food, including intense cravings and an inability to cut down on intake despite a desire to do so [43, 56]. Thus, many Americans would likely benefit from approaches to reduce the dominance of ultra-processed foods in the American food supply. Finally, another key point learned from the tobacco addiction epidemic is that prevention efforts can be far more cost effective than relying solely on treatment [57]. Targeting prevention efforts on youth, especially, can be particularly helpful to shape lifelong health promoting behaviors [57].

Eating is necessary for survival. We each make numerous food-related decisions every day all while surrounded by grocery stores, restaurants, gas stations, convenience stores and marketing that promote ultra-processed foods. It is essential that we address the factors that contribute to obesity and diabetes and encourage an American food supply that promotes health, particularly for our children.

**Table 1.** Diagnostic criteria for substance use disorders

| DSM–5 Diagnostic Criteria for Substance Use Disorders (30) |
|---|
| Consumption of larger amounts and/or over longer time than intended |
| Persistent, unsuccessful attempts to cut down |
| Significant time spent obtaining, using, or recovering from effects |
| Cravings (i.e., intense almost irresistible urges for the substance) |
| Interference with role obligations at work, school, or home |
| Use despite social or interpersonal problems |
| Important activities given up or reduced |
| Use in physically hazardous situations |
| Continued use despite physical and/or psychological consequences |
| Tolerance (i.e., needing more and more of the substance to get the desired effect) |
| Withdrawal (i.e., experiencing psychological and/or physiological symptoms when reducing intake) |

Individuals meet the diagnostic threshold for a substance use disorder in the Substance-Related and Addictive Disorders section of the Diagnostic and Statistical Manual of Mental Disorders-Fifth Edition (DSM 5) by endorsing at least 2 of the symptoms above plus clinically sig- nificant functional impairment or distress (30). Severity of substance use disorders determined by the number of symptoms endorsed (mild 2–3 symptoms; moderate 4–5 symptoms; severe 6–11 symptoms).

## References

[1] Sutton C. A., Stratton M., L'Insalata A. M., Fazzino TL. Ultraprocessed, hyper-palatable, and high energy density foods: Prevalence and distinction across 30 years in the United States. *Obesity*. 2023.

[2] Juul F., Parekh N., Martinez-Steele E., Monteiro C. A., Chang V. W. Ultra-processed food consumption among U.S. adults from 2001 to 2018. *The American Journal of Clinical Nutrition*. 2022;115(1):211–21.

[3] Scrinis G., Monteiro C. From ultra-processed foods to ultra-processed dietary patterns. *Nature Food*. 2022;3(9):671–3.

[4] Monteiro C. A., Cannon G., Levy R. B., Moubarac J-C., Louzada M. L., Rauber F., et al. Ultra-processed foods: what they are and how to identify them. *Public health nutrition*. 2019;22(5):936–41.

[5] Hall K. D.. From dearth to excess: the rise of obesity in an ultra-processed food system. *Philosophical Transactions of the Royal Society B*. 2023;378(1885):20220214.

[6] Steele E. M., Baraldi L. G., da Costa Louzada M. L., Moubarac J-C., Mozaffarian D, Monteiro CA. Ultra-processed foods and added sugars in the U.S. diet: evidence from a nationally representative cross-sectional study. *BMJ open.* 2016;6(3):e009892.

[7] Martinez Steele E., Popkin B. M., Swinburn B, Monteiro C. A. The share of ultra- processed foods and the overall nutritional quality of diets in the U.S.: evidence from a nationally representative cross-sectional study. *Population health metrics.* 2017;15:1–11.

[8] Fazzino T. L. The reinforcing natures of hyper-palatable foods: behavioral evidence for their reinforcing properties and the role of the U.S. food industry in promoting their availability. *Current Addiction Reports. 2022;9(4):298–306.*

[9] Wang L., Steele E. M., Du M., Pomeranz J. L., O'Connor L. E., Herrick K. A., et al. Trends in consumption of ultraprocessed foods among U.S. youths aged 2–19 years, 1999–2018. *Jama.* 2021;326(6):519–30.

[10] Touvier M., da Costa Louzada M. L., Mozaffarian D, Baker P, Juul F, Srour B. Ultra-processed foods and cardiometabolic health: public health policies to reduce consumption cannot wait. *bmj.* 2023;383.

[11] Hall K. D., Ayuketah A., Brychta R., Cai H., Cassimatis T., Chen K. Y., et al. Ultra- processed diets cause excess calorie intake and weight gain: an inpatient randomized controlled trial of ad libitum food intake. *Cell metabolism.* 2019;30(1):67–77. e3.

[12] Chen Z., Khandpur N., Desjardins C., Wang L., Monteiro C. A., Rossato S. L., et al. Ultra-processed food consumption and risk of type 2 diabetes: three large prospective U.S. cohort studies. *Diabetes Care.* 2023;46(7):1335–44.

[13] Gearhardt A. N., DiFeliceantonio A. G.. Highly processed foods can be considered addictive substances based on established scientific criteria. *Addiction.* 2022.

[14] Nelson R. A., Boyd S. J., Ziegelstein R. C., Herning R., Cadet J. L., Henningfield J. E., et al. Effect of rate of administration on subjective and physiological effects of intravenous cocaine in humans. *Drug and alcohol dependence.* 2006;82(1):19–24.

[15] De Wit H., Bodker B., Ambre J. Rate of increase of plasma drug level influences subjective response in humans. *Psychopharmacology.* 1992;107:352–8.

[16] Heinz A., Daedelow L. S., Wackerhagen C, Di Chiara G. Addiction theory matters—why there is no dependence on caffeine or antidepressant medication. *Addiction Biology.* 2020;25(2):e12735.

[17] Robinson T. E., Berridge K. C.. Incentive-sensitization and addiction. *Addiction.* 2001;96(11177523):103–14.

[18] DeCicca P., Kenkel D., Liu F, Somerville J. Quantifying brand loyalty: evidence from the cigarette market. *Journal of health economics.* 2021;79:102512.

[19] Rose J. E., Salley A., Behm F. M., Bates JE, Westman E. C. Reinforcing effects of nicotine and non-nicotine components of cigarette smoke. *Psychopharmacology.* 2010;210:1–12.

[20] West R., Cox S. The 1988 U.S. Surgeon General's report 'Nicotine Addiction': How well has it stood up to three more decades of research? *Addiction.* 2022;117(8):2346–50.

[21] Gearhardt A. N., Bueno N. B., DiFeliceantonio AG, Roberto CA, Jiminez-Murcia S, Fernandez-Aranda F. Social, clinical, and policy implications of ultra-processed food addiction. *bmj.* 2023;383.

[22] DiFeliceantonio A. G., Coppin G, Rigoux L., Thanarajah S. E., Dagher A., Tittgemeyer M., et al. Supra-additive effects of combining fat and carbohydrate on food reward. *Cell metabolism.* 2018;28(1):33–44. e3.

[23] Ahmed SH, Guillem K, Vandaele Y. Sugar addiction: pushing the drug-sugar analogy to the limit. Current Opinion in Clinical Nutrition & Metabolic *Care.* 2013;16(4):434–9.

[24] Di Chiara G., Imperato A. Drugs abused by humans preferentially increase synaptic dopamine concentrations in the mesolimbic system of freely moving rats. *Proceedings of the National Academy of Sciences.* 1988;85(14):5274–8.

[25] Bassareo V., De Luca M. A., Aresu M., Aste A., Ariu T., Di Chiara G. Differential adaptive properties of accumbens shell dopamine responses to ethanol as a drug and as a motivational stimulus. *European Journal of Neuroscience.* 2003;17(7):1465–72.

[26] Hajnal A., Smith G. P., Norgren R. Oral sucrose stimulation increases accumbens dopamine in the rat. *American Journal of Physiology-Regulatory, Integrative and Comparative Physiology.* 2004;286(1):R31-R7.

[27] Bassareo V., Di Chiara G. Differential influence of associative and nonassociative learning mechanisms on the responsiveness of prefrontal and accumbal dopamine transmission to food stimuli in rats fed ad libitum. *Journal of Neuroscience.* 1997;17(2):851–61.

[28] Bassareo V., De Luca M. A., Di Chiara G. Differential expression of motivational stimulus properties by dopamine in nucleus accumbens shell versus core and prefrontal cortex. *Journal of neuroscience.* 2002;22(11):4709–19.

[29] De Luca M. A. Habituation of the responsiveness of mesolimbic and mesocortical dopamine transmission to taste stimuli. *Frontiers in integrative neuroscience.* 2014;8:21.

[30] American Psychiatric Association. Diagnostic and statistical manual of mental disorders (DSM–5): American Psychiatric Pub; 2013.

[31] Gearhardt A. N., Corbin W. R., Brownell K. D. Preliminary validation of the Yale Food Addiction Scale. Appetite. 2009;52:430–6.

[32] Gearhardt AN, Schulte EM. Is food addictive? A review of the science. *Annual Review of Nutrition.* 2021;41:387–410.

[33] Schulte E. M., Avena N. M., Gearhardt AN. Which foods may be addictive? The roles of processing, fat content, and glycemic load. *PloS one.* 2015;10(2):e0117959.

[34] Schulte E. M., Smeal JK, Gearhardt A. N. Foods are differentially associated with subjective effect report questions of abuse liability. *PLoS One.* 2017;12(8):e0184220.

[35] Leung C. W., Parnarouskis L, Slotnick M. J., Gearhardt A. N. Food insecurity and food addiction in a large, national sample of lower-income adults. *Current Developments in Nutrition.* 2023:102036.

[36] Whatnall M., Clarke E., Collins C. E., Pursey K, Burrows T. Ultra-processed food intakes associated with 'food addiction in young adults. *Appetite.* 2022;178:106260.

[37] Filgueiras A. R., de Almeida V. B. P., Nogueira P. C. K., Domene S. M. A., da Silva CE, Sesso R, et al. Exploring the consumption of ultra-processed foods and its association with food addiction in overweight children. *Appetite.* 2019;135:137–45.

[38] Praxedes D. R., Silva-Junior AE, Macena ML, Oliveira AD, Cardoso KS, Nunes LO, et al. Prevalence of food addiction determined by the Yale Food Addiction Scale and associated factors: A systematic review with meta-analysis. *European Eating Disorders Review.* 2022;30(2):85–95.

[39] Grant B. F., Dawson D. A., Stinson F. S., Chou S. P., Dufour MC, Pickering RP. The 12-month prevalence and trends in DSM-IV alcohol abuse and dependence: United States, 1991—1992 and 2001—2002. *Drug and alcohol dependence.* 2004;74(3):223–34.

[40] Organization WH. *WHO report on the global tobacco epidemic, 2019: offer help to quit tobacco use: World Health Organization*; 2019.

[41] Horsager C., Bruun J. M., Furk E., Hagstr m S, Lauritsen MB, stergaard SD. Food Addiction is Strongly Associated With Type 2 Diabetes. *Clinical Nutrition.* 2023.

[42] Yekaninejad M. S., Badrooj N., Vosoughi F., Lin C. Y., Potenza M. N., Pakpour A. H. Prevalence of food addiction in children and adolescents: A systematic review and meta-analysis. *Obesity Reviews.* 2021;22(6):e13183.

[43] Kullgren J, Solway E, Roberts S, Gearhardt A, Singer D, Kirch M, et al. *National Poll on Healthy Aging: Addiction to Highly Processed Food Among Older Adults.* 2023.

[44] LaFata E. M., Gearhardt A. N. Ultra-Processed Food Addiction: An Epidemic? *Psychotherapy and Psychosomatics.* 2022;91(6):363–72.
[45] Nguyen K. H., Glantz S. A, Palmer C. N., Schmidt L. A. Transferring racial/ethnic marketing strategies from tobacco to food corporations: Philip Morris and Kraft General Foods. *American journal of public health.* 2020;110(3):329–36.
[46] Nguyen K. H., Glantz S. A., Palmer C. N., Schmidt LA. Tobacco industry involvement in children's sugary drinks market. *BMJ.* 2019;364.
[47] Fazzino T. L., Jun D., Chollet-Hinton L, Bjorlie K. U.S. tobacco companies selectively disseminated hyper-palatable foods into the U.S. food system: Empirical evidence and current implications. *Addiction.* 2023.
[48] Selvin E., Parrinello C. M., Sacks D. B., Coresh J. Trends in prevalence and control of diabetes in the United States, 1988—1994 and 1999—2010. *Annals of internal medicine.* 2014;160(8):517–25.
[49] Gregg E. W., Cheng Y. J., Narayan K. V., Thompson TJ, Williamson DF. The relative contributions of different levels of overweight and obesity to the increased prevalence of diabetes in the United States: 1976—2004. *Preventive medicine.* 2007;45(5):348–52.
[50] Robinson J. H., Pritchard WS. The role of nicotine in tobacco use. *Psychopharmacology.* 1992;108:397–407.
[51] Henningfield J. E., Keenan R. M. Nicotine delivery kinetics and abuse liability. *J. Consult Clin Psychol.* 1993;61(8245272):743–50.
[52] Warner K. E. Policy Lessons Learned from Tobacco. *Food and Addiction: A Comprehensive Handbook.* 2012;416.
[53] Warner K. E, Mendez D. Tobacco control policy in developed countries: yesterday, today, and tomorrow. *Nicotine & Tobacco Research.* 2010;12(9):876–87.
[54] Warner K. E., Tam J. The impact of tobacco control research on policy: 20 years of progress. *Tobacco control.* 2012;21(2):103–9.
[55] McLellan A. T., Koob G. F., Volkow ND. Preaddiction—A Missing Concept for Treating Substance Use Disorders. *JAMA psychiatry.* 2022.
[56] Schulte E. M., Gearhardt ANJEEDR. Associations of food addiction in a sample recruited to be nationally representative of the United States. 2018;26(2):112–9.
[57] Miller T. R., Hendrie D. Substance abuse prevention dollars and cents: A cost- benefit analysis: U.S. Department of Health and Human Services, *Substance Abuse and Mental*; 2009.

## Summary Statement of Ashley Gearhardt

*Ultra-Processed Foods Dominate the American Diet:* The American diet is now composed mostly of ultra-processed foods, which are industrial formulations manufactured by deconstructing foods into their component parts, modifying them and recombining them with a myriad of additives. The average American now gets most of their calories from ultra-processed foods and they are major sources of added sugar and saturated fats. Ultra-processed foods are implicated in health conditions like depression and obesity. Every 10 percent increase in ultra-processed food intake is associated with a 12 percent higher risk of Type 2 diabetes.

*There are Strong Parallels between Addictive Substances and Ultra-Processed Foods:* Addictive substances are created through processing natural substances to rapidly deliver unnaturally high doses of reinforcing ingredients to the body. Ultra-processed foods are created by altering natural substances into products that deliver unnaturally high doses of carbohydrates and fat, which are rapidly absorbed. This activates the reward systems implicated in addiction. Additives further enhance the flavor and texture of these products.

*Key Signs of Addiction Occur in the Intake of Ultra-Processed Food:* Systematic reviews of over 280 studies estimate that 14 percent of adults and 12 percent of children meet the criteria for an addictive disorder in their intake of ultraprocessed foods. This prevalence is doubled in individuals with obesity. This addictive pattern of ultra-processed food intake is associated with a more than five times greater likelihood of Type 2 diabetes. If addictive mechanisms are being triggered by ultra-processed foods, this may be an overlooked reason why it can be challenging to reduce their intake even in the face of health conditions like diabetes.

*There are Strong Connections between the Tobacco and Processed Food Industries*: From the 1980's to the late 2000's, tobacco companies like RJ Reynolds and Philip Morris became the biggest producers of processed food in the world. Internal tobacco industry documents demonstrate strategies designed to develop and sell cigarettes were applied to processed food products, such as adding flavor additives developed for cigarettes into children's sugar-sweetened beverages and targeting children and racial/ethnic minorities in marketing.

*Lessons Learned from the Tobacco Epidemic Can Guide Solutions:* Investing in science to understand how ultra-processed food activate mechanisms of addiction and contribute to excessive intake is important.

Multi-pronged approaches and a focus on prevention, particularly for youth, will be important for improving American's health.

The CHAIR. Thank you very much, Dr. Gearhardt. Our next witness will be Dr. Lindsey Smith Taillie, Associate Professor in the Department of Nutrition at the University of North Carolina at Chapel Hill.

Dr. Taillie is a nutrition epidemiologist who evaluates food policies and the industry's influence on consumer choices. Dr. Taillie, thanks so much for being with us.

## Statement of Lindsey Smith Taillie, Ph.D., Associate Professor, Department of Nutrition, University of North Carolina, Chapel Hill, NC

Dr. TAILLIE. Chairman Sanders, Ranking Member Cassidy, and distinguished Members of the Committee, thank you for the opportunity to speak with you.

My name is Lindsey Smith Taillie, and I am in nutrition epidemiologist who works in the U.S. and globally. My research focuses on understanding how the food industry and the food environment influences nutrition, particularly among kids, as well as what policies work to create healthier diets.

In every country where I work, one thing is true, parents want to make healthy choices for their kids. However, the current food environment makes it nearly impossible. Diets are a major driver of obesity and type 2 diabetes, and this problem is especially alarming for kids. In the U.S., pediatric type 2 diabetes has doubled over the last two decades.

Healthier diets prevent diabetes and are more cost effective than medication. So why don't we change our diet? First, our food supply. Most of our packaged foods are ultra-processed and nearly half are too high in added sugar, sodium, and saturated fat.

Our food contains more sugar and sweeteners than other high income countries. We can't make healthy choices if healthy food is unavailable. Second, these products are aggressively marketed to children and disproportionately targeted to black and Hispanic youth. Food companies spend $14 billion a year on food advertising in the U.S., of which 80 percent is for unhealthy foods.

Marketing is powerful. It makes kids want unhealthy foods, and it makes them consume more of them. Third, kids will get mostly ultra-processed foods at school. Unhealthy food marketing inside schools is also very common. This serves to hook kids on unhealthy foods at a very early age. It is also very hard for parents to know what is healthy versus unhealthy. Nutrition claims like 100 percent all natural are very common in our food supply and lend an aura of helpfulness even to unhealthy foods.

Meanwhile, the Nutrition Facts panel provides useful information but can be hard to understand. Parents can't make informed choices without accessible information. Another major factor is price. Ultra-processed foods tend to be cheaper than healthy foods.

Even though parents want to buy healthy foods, they buy ultra- processed because it is cheaper. Right now, the price of these unhealthy products does not reflect the health cost of consuming them. Last, the food industry has interfered with science and policy. Companies that pay to play by funding professional societies and research scientists to change the narrative about what causes obesity and diabetes.

They also position themselves as part of the solution through voluntary initiatives, despite overwhelming scientific evidence that these programs are ineffective. So how can we fix this? We already have good data on what works. First, the U.S. should require clear nutrition labels on the front of food packages, a policy that the majority of Americans support across political parties.

The FDA is currently researching front of package labels for the U.S. However, many of the designs that the FDA is focusing on are not based on the scientific evidence from the 10 countries that have implemented these labels, nor the many experiments we have conducted in the U.S.

For example, several of the proposed FDA labels include numbers or color schemes that research shows consumers do not understand. In contrast, simple nutrient warnings like those in Mexico and most of South America are well understood even by children. In addition, in countries with these labels, the food industry has cut sugar, sodium, and saturated fat with no adverse effect on the economy.

The FDA needs to work closely with scientists to develop evidence backed labels that are easy to understand and clearly signal to consumers when products are unhealthy. Second, the U.S. should limit unhealthy food marketing to kids, much as it has for tobacco. Restricting where ads appear and the use of techniques like cartoons cut kids exposure and helps them develop healthy preferences.

Also, companies should not be allowed to take tax deductions on what they spend on food advertising. Third, our kids deserve classrooms that are free from corporate food. We should restrict the marketing, promotion, and sale of ultra-processed foods in schools, which global data show reduces their availability and improves children's diets.

We also should use economic pressure to shift the food supply. Just like in tobacco, poor diets create massive health care burden and health costs in the U.S. And as in tobacco, taxes on the production of sugary drinks and ultra-processed foods would make food companies pay the true cost of these products.

Global data show that these taxes spur companies to create healthier products and reduce the consumption of unhealthy foods. To further support diabetes prevention, revenue from these taxes could be used to fund fruits and vegetables subsidies for low income families. Last, we need more funding for nutrition research.

Even though nutrition is the leading cause of obesity and diabetes, only a tiny fraction of the NIH budget goes toward nutrition. Additional research funding is critical to improving diets and preventing obesity and diabetes.

In conclusion, kids should not be sick because of our food environment. Federal policy action is urgently needed to make the healthy choice the easy choice. Thank you.

[The prepared statement of Dr. Taillie follows:]

## Prepared Statement of Lindsey Smith Taillie

Chairman Sanders, Ranking Member Cassidy, and Members of the Committee:

My name is Lindsey Smith Taillie, and I am an associate professor of nutrition and nutrition epidemiologist. I appreciate the opportunity to speak with you today about my research on how the food industry and food environments influence nutrition, obesity, and type 2 diabetes, as well as policy actions that other countries are using to address these issues.

For the last decade, I have worked in the United States and many countries in Latin America, Africa, and Asia to research the design and test the effectiveness of food policies. Our goal has been to create a toolkit for what works to prevent the continued increase in diet-related chronic diseases. Our premise, backed by scientific evidence, is that consumers want to make healthier choices, but that the current food environment makes it nearly impossible for them to do so.

*First, obesity and diabetes are pressing public health concerns.* Twenty percent of our children have obesity, as do 42 percent of American adults (Hu & Staiano 2022; Li 2022). Obesity is linked to a plethora of adverse health effects, including sleep apnea, joint pain, cardiovascular disease, cancer, and type 2 diabetes (Wang 2019; Raud 2020; Larsson 2019; Pati 2023; Klein 2022). Even more concerning, the incidence of type 2 diabetes among children has nearly doubled over the last 20 years (Wagenknecht 2023). These problems do not impact all Americans equally—Black and Hispanic children have been disproportionately affected, with steeper increases in both obesity and diabetes (Katz, Rodriguez & Knowles 2021). These health consequences are also very costly: Over $300 billion dollars is spent annually in the U.S. to treat diabetes, with an additional $100 billion spent on indirect costs like lower work productivity, unemployment due to chronic disability, and premature death (Parker 2023). About 67 percent of diabetes costs are paid by Medicare and Medicaid (U.S. Department of Health and Human Services 2021).

*Poor diets are the culprit of the obesity and type 2 diabetes epidemics.* Americans are the world's leading consumers of sugary drinks and ultraprocessed foods. Put simply, ultraprocessed foods are what you might know as "junk food:" food that is industrially produced and often contains high levels of added sugar, sodium, and saturated fat, as well as additives, colorants, and preservatives. Currently, approximately half of American children and adults consume sugary drinks on a given day (Marriott 2019). Drinking sugary beverages promotes excess calorie intake, which leads to weight gain (Nguyen 2023). Over time, the accumulation of fat can turn into non-alcoholic fatty liver disease, increase risk of diabetes, and raise the risk of heart disease (Qin 2020; Chen 2019; Yang 2022). Relevant to this hearing, obesity contributes to the development of type 2 diabetes by promoting insulin resistance, inflammation, and dysfunction of insulin-producing cells (Kahn 2016; Luca & Olefsky 2008). In other words, excess fat disrupts our bodies' ability to produce and use insulin. Research also suggests that unhealthy diets can increase cardiometabolic risk through other mechanisms like altering the gut microbiome, disrupting hormonal signaling pathways, and affecting the brain's reward responses (Stanhope 2018).

Ultraprocessed foods also pose a major threat to our health. A century ago, ultraprocessed foods did not exist. Now, 57 percent of calories consumed by U.S. adults and 67 percent of calories consumed by kids come from ultraprocessed foods (Juul 2022; Wang 2021), with consumption rising most rapidly among Black and Mexican youths (Wang 2021). High consumption of ultraprocessed foods substantially increases risk of obesity (Moradi 2023; Lane 2020), metabolic syndrome (Lane 2020), and cardiovascular disease (Suksatan 2022). The most compelling evidence to date comes from a rigorous randomized crossover trial conducted by Kevin Hall at the NIH (Hall 2021). In the study, participants were allowed to eat freely from nutrient-matched ultraprocessed vs. minimally processed menus for 2 weeks. The study found that during the ultraprocessed weeks, participants consumed roughly 500 more calories/day and gained 2.2 lbs (of mostly fat mass).

Sugary drinks and ultraprocessed foods are designed for overconsumption, leading people to take in more calories than they want or realize. It is very easy to overconsume ultraprocessed foods because they are ''hyperpalatable,'' meaning they combine salty, sweet, and fat flavors in irresistible combinations not found in nature. They do not require much time or effort to prepare and are often eaten on the go or in front of a computer or TV, making it easy to eat or drink more than we realize. On a chemical level, ultraprocessed food ingredients are degraded to the point that they no longer give us feelings of fullness during digestion and send sugar and fat into our bloodstream more quickly.

Improving diets could prevent and delay the onset of type 2 diabetes in a way that is more effective and cheaper than medication (Lee 2019; CHOICES). The Diabetes Prevention Program clinical trial found better diets and physical activity reduced incidence of diabetes by 58 percent compared with a placebo, while metformin reduced incidence by 31 percent (Diab Prev Program Research Group 2002).

Consumers want to make healthy choices. However, it is very difficult to eat healthy diets in the current American food environment for the following reasons:

- *Food supply:* The U.S. food supply is rife with unhealthy foods: 50 percent of U.S. packaged foods in 2020 were ultraprocessed, while 43 percent were high in sugar, sodium, or saturated fat (under review). The U.S. has more sugar and non-caloric sweeteners in its packaged food supply compared to other high-income, English-speaking countries (Dunford 2018), and we consume on average 73 pounds of sugar, corn syrup, and other sweeteners per year (USDA 2023). Product-for-product, our food supply is sweeter: for example, the sugar content in children's breakfast cereals is 10–20 percent higher than in comparable countries (Chepulis 2019). The U.S. food supply is also full of industrial food additives (e.g., colors, flavors, flavor enhancers, emulsifiers, thickeners, and artificial sweeteners)—ingredients which are added to make the products more palatable and increase consumption. As of 2019, nearly 60 percent of U.S. consumer food purchases—and alarmingly, 73 percent of baby food purchases—contained additives (Dunford 2023).

- *Food marketing*: Sugary drinks and ultraprocessed foods are aggressively marketed to children. Food companies spend roughly $14 billion per year on food advertising in the U.S., of which 80 percent is for unhealthy foods (Rudd Center Food Marketing 2023). Companies target children with marketing for unhealthy foods everywhere they live, learn, and play, including on TV, social media, in product placement, at school, and on their toys and clothing, and by using tactics like licensed characters, A green and black television celebrities, games, spokespeople, contests, and kids' clubs to attract their attention. Targeted marketing to children is very common: every day, U.S. children see an estimated 10 ads for unhealthy foods on TV alone (Fleming-Milici 2017). Advertising to youth is shifting from television to digital and mobile platforms, including ads on social media, branded games and ordering apps, and paid promotions from bloggers, influencers, and brand Ambassadors—marketing that is often disguised as entertainment. For example, teenagers see food marketing 189 times per week on social media apps—most for unhealthy foods (Potvin Kent 2019). Children are uniquely vulnerable to the impact of food marketing because of their inability to recognize its persuasive intent (Harris 2009). This exposure to unhealthy food and beverage advertisements increases youth's preference, selection, and consumption of unhealthy foods (Tsochantaridou 2023; Norman 2016).
- It is also very concerning that food companies target unhealthy food marketing specifically to youth of color, who are most at risk for diabetes. For example, fast food and sugary drink ads appear at a higher rate on Spanish-language TV than English language TV; schools with > 60 percent Hispanic populations have more outdoor food and beverage ads within a half a mile of the school (CSPI 2023). Food companies target children of color by designing specific products for them, adapting pricing, advertising on specific channels or in places in the community, using their own language and cultural

references, and personalizing digital advertisements. Companies do this because children of color represent a rapidly growing market with significant economic impact, have high levels of media use, and are trend-setters for the general public. For example, marketing campaigns targeting youth of color use cause-related marketing like donations or collaborations with non-profits. Coca Cola and Pepsi are responsible for the majority of these marketing campaigns and they almost exclusively promote unhealthy foods (Rudd Center Targeted Marketing).

- *Food prices*: Cost drives food purchasing decisions, and unhealthy foods tend to be cheaper than healthy foods. For example, in New York City, the price per liter of sugary drinks is higher than low-calorie drinks (Bragg 2022). In many parts of the world, sugary drinks are cheaper than water (Blecher 2017); ultraprocessed foods also have lower per-calorie cost and have faced slower price increases in recent years (Gupta 2019). Low-income people are more affected and report having to purchase ultraprocessed foods and snacks vs. fruits and vegetables due to price (Ravikumar 2022).
- *Labeling*: The current food labeling environment is very confusing to consumers. Nutrition-related claims on food packages are very common (Taillie 2018; USDA 2023); yet their presence does not reliably indicate that a product is actually healthy. For example, 97 percent of fruit drinks, the top-consumed sugary drink among kids, carry some type of claim like ''100 percent Vitamin C'' or ''Natural'' (Duffy 2021). These claims lead to the ''health halo'' effect, in which claims give unhealthy products an aura of healthfulness, leading parents to make less healthy choices (Hall 2023; Hall 2020). The Nutrition Facts Panel got important updates in 2020, including the requirement to disclose added sugar content. However, few consumers consistently use these back-of-the package labels, with low-income and low-educated populations less likely to use them (Storz 2023). Moreover, people spend only seconds selecting a food item, making it difficult to understand complex, numeric information and make educated decisions.
- *School foods*: Kids consume about a third of their daily calories at school; foods served and sold to children in schools also affect lifetime food preferences. The Healthy, Hunger Free Kids Act improved the nutritional quality of school foods and helped prevent

obesity among children in poverty, with no difference in school meal participation (Johnson 2016; Kenney 2020). However, our team's analyses of National Health and Nutrition Survey data found that in 2015–2018, the majority of calories kids consume at school comes from ultraprocessed foods (Vatavuk, unpublished). Moreover, unhealthy food marketing is highly prevalent in schools, with companies providing school sports sponsorships, student in centives (e.g., Pizza Hut's Book It program), branded fundraising and reward programs (e.g., General Mill's Box Tops for Education; fast food proceed donations), digital and physical advertisements, and the sales of branded fast-food products (Harris 2014). In addition, ''Smart Snacks,'' or packaged snacks that have been reformulated to meet USDA school foods standards, are virtually indistinguishable from the less healthy versions sold outside of schools (Harris 2016). Thus, even these ''healthier'' snacks serve as another form of marketing to get kids hooked on specific brands, increasing their preferences and purchases.

- *Food retail environment:* Sugary drinks and ultraprocessed foods are ubiquitous in all retail settings and are often at checkouts, at endcaps of stores and are often placed in locations and heights that children are more likely to see and pester their parents to get. For example, a national study found 91 percent of supermarkets carry candy at checkout and 85 percent carry sugary drinks (Barker 2015).
- *Corporate interference:* To circumvent regulation, the food industry has followed the tobacco industry playbook: blaming personal responsibility, casting doubt on unfavorable research, funding favorable research, coopting professional organizations, lobbying, and arguing for self-regulation (Stuckler & Nestle 2012). For example, the sugar and sugary drinks industry has sought to shift the blame from sugar to fat (Kearns 2016); created a shadow group to create allies in academia and governments for pro-sugar policies, funded physical activity research to change the narrative about what causes obesity (Serodio 2018), and funded major nutrition and health societies in exchange for influence over proceedings (e.g., the American Academy of Nutrition and Dietetics) (Gunnarsson 2022).
- The packaged food industry has proposed voluntary labeling and marketing self-regulations in an attempt to circumvent regulation. However, these initiatives have failed: they are slow, ineffective, and

contain many loopholes while allowing companies to claim to be part of the solution (Boyland 2022). Federal regulation is needed to create healthier food environments. Many countries, particularly in Latin America, have already begun taking action. Below, I outline evidence-based policy recommendations to promote healthier diets and prevent diet-related diseases.

## Key Recommendations

### 1. Require Front-of-Package Labels on Unhealthy Foods

Since 2016, 10 countries have mandated front-of-package nutrition labels on foods high in sugar, sodium, and saturated fat, which includes all sugary drinks and most ultraprocessed foods. Compared to other labeling systems, ''high-in'' labels that signal when a product is high in unhealthy nutrients more effectively empower consumers to avoid nutrients of concern (Croker 2020). A simple black-and-white design grabs consumers' attention and is easily understood, even by children and those with limited English proficiency (Correa 2019; Hall 2021). Chile was the first country to implement high-in labels, leading to a 24 percent drop in sugary drink purchases and a 24 percent drop in purchases of foods carrying the labels (Taillie 2020, 2021). Chile's policy also incentivized the food industry to cut sugar and sodium in the food supply (Reyes 2020), with no adverse impacts on wages and employment (Paraje 2023). Many countries have followed Chile's lead and implemented similar warning label regulations—covering much of South America as well as Mexico and Canada. The FDA is currently researching front-of-package labeling options for the U.S. and plans to issue a proposed regulation requiring new labels in June 2024. FDA should consider that single-nutrient octagonal labels maximize consumers' ability to quickly and accurately identify unhealthy products, more so than labels with numerical information requiring numeracy skills (Grummon 2019). Ample experimental research in the U.S. already shows that warning labels help consumers quickly identify unhealthy foods and make healthier, informed choices (Musicus 2023; Taillie 2022). Using evidence-supported visuals like icons or symbols further increases comprehension (Hall 2021; Bopape 2021). Most importantly, the FDA must ensure that progress toward clear, informative labeling is led by governments and public health experts, not commercial interests.

1a. FOP labels should include visuals to increase comprehension, use single-nutrient octagonal labels to maximize consumers' ability to quickly and accurately identify products high in nutrients of concern (including sugar), and avoid including information about the percent of the daily value ( percent DV).

1b. Restaurants should require similar labels. In November 2023, New York City passed the ''Sweet Truth Act'' that will require chains with 15 or more restaurants to use an added sugar icon on their menus and menu boards to indicate a food or drink item contains more than 50g of added sugar.

## 2. Restrict Food Marketing to Children

Policies to reduce children's exposure to harmful food marketing should protect children of all ages (up to age 18 years); use a strong, government-led nutrient profiling to classify foods for restriction; be comprehensive enough to minimize the risk of migration of marketing to other media or to other age groups; and restrict the persuasive power of food marketing (World Health Organization, 2023). Chile provides the most compelling example of the impacts a strong marketing policy. In 2016, Chile restricted the use of child-directed appeals on products exceeding set nutrient thresholds, restricted placement of ads in media with high child viewership, and prohibited the sales and promotion of these products in school. In 2018, they extended this regulation by banning television advertisements on unhealthy food advertisement between 6am-10pm. Together, these regulations have worked in a relatively short amount of time to dramatically reduce children's exposure to unhealthy food marketing and lessen its persuasive appeal and power:

- In the first (and most lenient) year of the law, the percentage of TV ads for foods and drinks high in energy, saturated fats, sugars, or sodium dropped from 42 percent to 15 percent (Correa 2020).
- By 2019, Chile's marketing restrictions led to a total drop of 73 percent in children's daily exposure to TV ads for products high in calories, sugar, salt or saturated fat on all TV and a 90 percent drop during children's programming (Dillman Carpentier 2023). What's more, 67 percent fewer unhealthy food ads on TV used child-directed creative content such as cartoons, characters, toys, or contests, which are also prohibited under the country's laws.

- The percentage of regulated cereals (typically high in calories and/or sugar) with child-directed strategies featured on their packages dropped from 43 percent to 15 percent in the first year of regulation (Mediano Stolze et al. 2019).

### 3. Amend the Tax Code to Remove the Deductibility of Expenses Associated with Advertising and Marketing Foods and Beverages of Poor Nutritional Quality to Children

Food companies can deduct expenditures related to advertising and marketing from their taxes. Through this process, the U.S. government provides a subsidy for marketing unhealthy food and drinks to children (Center for Science in the Public Interest [CSPI] 2023). Removing the deductibility of advertising expenses on sugary drinks and ultraprocessed foods would incentivize companies to decrease unhealthy food marketing to children and could raise $80 million in Federal revenue annually (CSPI 2023).

### 4. Implement Taxes on Sugary Drinks and Ultraprocessed Foods and Subsidies on Healthier Foods

Tax policies would require legislative action and there have been several bills introduced to the U.S. Congress in recent years. We strongly recommend that a Federal tax on sugary drinks as proposed in the 2021 ''SWEET Act'' Bill, which sets a 2-cents/ounce tax on ready-to-drink lower- sugar SSBs and a 3-cents/ounce tax on ready-to-drink high-sugar SSBs. Importantly, it also proposes directing the resultant revenue toward public health and health promotion objectives. Uses of the revenue could include: improving school feeding programs and/or funding expansion of healthy incentive programs to support low-income families afford healthy foods as proposed in 2023 ''GusNIP Expansion Act'' and the ''Opt for Health with SNAP (OH SNAP) Close the Fruit and Vegetable Gap Act'' that were con-currently introduced into the U.S. House of Representatives and Senate, respectively. Dedicating the tax revenues toward lower-income communities and families would enhance the equity potential, with multiplier effects for the local economies of these families, and address concerns around the income regressivity of the tax. In a new modeling study, our team found that a tax on sugary drinks following the SWEET Act would lower calories purchased, while targeted subsidies would increase fruit, vegetable, and healthier drink purchases without substantially increasing calories (Pourya under review). A broader tax that also includes ultra-processed foods along with targeted subsidies for minimally processed foods could promote healthier food choices among low-income households and could be budget neutral for the Federal Government.

U.S. and global data show that sugary drink taxes reduce consumption (Andreyeva 2022; Teng 2019; Powell 2021), reduce sugar content in the food supply (Dickson 2023), and result in health benefits, including reduced pediatric hospital admissions from dental caries (Rogers 2023), and decreased prevalence of overweight and obesity, particularly where price increases are steeper (Gracner 2022). Modeling studies have predicted that in Mexico, where the first sugary drinks tax was implemented, the tax will lead to a 2.5 percent reduction in obesity prevalence and prevent 86 to 134 thousand cases of diabetes a decade after the tax (Barrientos 2017). Fewer data are available on foods taxes, but our research in Mexico found that a modest 8 percent junk food tax reduced taxed food purchases by ?5 percent (Batis 2016).

### 5. Incorporate Guidance on Ultraprocessed Foods into Dietary Guidelines

Increasingly, other countries (most recently, Mexico) include specific dietary guidance around the consumption of ultraprocessed foods. The 2025 U.S. Dietary Guidelines Advisory Committee is currently reviewing evidence on ultraprocessed foods for the 2025 Dietary Guidelines. Inclusion of guidance on ultraprocessed foods could help guide consumers and underpin other policies, including school foods.

### 6. Create Healthier School Environments

Schools should be a place where children can eat healthy foods and learn good nutrition, free from the influence of corporate marketing. Creating this environment will promote healthier diets that track into adulthood.

6a. Ideally, schools should not sell any foods that are high in added sugar or any nutrient of concern (as identified by the FOP warning labels in Recommendation 1). At a minimum, school lunch standards should follow the Dietary Guidelines and ensure that added sugars are limited to 10 percent of calories per week. Schools should have product-based limits for high-sugar foods, including grain-based desserts, breakfast cereals, yogurts, and flavored milks, as well as other products like condiments, toppings, and dressings. Schools should not offer flavored sweetened milk, particularly among young children (under grade 9). We applaud many of the USDA's proposed updates to school nutrition standards which would address several of these concerns. The USDA could go even further by considering a policy like Brazil's, which requires that 75 percent of school food procurement expenditures be used on fresh or minimally processed foods, with only 20 percent allowed for purchasing processed and ultraprocessed foods.

6b. School food environments should be free from advertising, promotions, and marketing of products high in nutrients of concern. Again, Chile serves as an example: after banning the sales and promotion of unhealthy foods in schools, availability of unhealthy foods dropped from 97 percent of foods and 76 percent of beverages to only 14 percent, with concurrent reductions in calories, saturated fats, sodium, and sugar available to purchase (Massri 2019). After the policies, Chilean children consumed significantly less total sugar at school (Fretes 2021).

## 6. Increase Nutrition Funding

A major barrier to progress in using nutrition to prevent diabetes is lack of scientific funding, which has remained flat over decades (Fleischhacker 2020). The National Institutes of Health only spends ?5 percent of its annual budget on nutrition, with only 1.3 percent dedicated to understanding the role of diet in preventing or treating disease. Increased funding for nutrition science is critical for preventing obesity, diabetes, and other diet-related chronic diseases.

Ideally, multiple of these policies would be implemented together as a policy package. Our experiences with food policies implemented in many countries suggest an interactive and reinforcing effect. For example, front-of-package nutrition labels can be used to guide what is permissible to market and sell in schools, where children can further learn how to use the labels to tell what is healthy vs. not healthy. Together, these policies can create healthier food environments for children, promoting healthier dietary behaviors that track into adulthood and help prevent obesity, type 2 diabetes, and other diet-related chronic diseases across the lifecycle.

## Summary Statement of Lindsey Smith Taillie

Why diet matters for type 2 diabetes prevention:

- The U.S. has an alarmingly high prevalence of obesity and type 2 diabetes. The incidence of type 2 diabetes among children has doubled over the last 20 years, with Black and Hispanic children experiencing the fastest increases.
- Americans consume too much sugary drinks and ultraprocessed foods. Often known as ''junk food,'' ultraprocessed foods are industrially produced foods that typically contain additives and high levels of added sugar, sodium, saturated fat, and excessive calories. Nearly 2/3 of kids' daily calories come from ultraprocessed foods, and the steepest increases have occurred among Black and Hispanic youth.
- Sugary drinks and ultraprocessed foods lead to weight gain, which promotes diabetes. In an NIH trial, just 2 weeks on an ultraprocessed food diet led people to consume ?500 more calories per day and gain weight.
- Sugary drinks and ultraprocessed foods are designed for overconsumption because they combine flavors, sugar, salt, and fat in ways not found in nature; they are cheap; they are convenient; and we digest them more quickly.
- Improving diet quality would prevent and delay onset of type 2 diabetes and is more cost-effective than medication.

The U.S. food environment makes it very difficult for Americans to make healthy choices.

- Food supply: The U.S. food supply contains more sugar and sweeteners than other high-income countries. Fifty percent of U.S. packaged foods are ultraprocessed and 43 percent are high in sugar, sodium, or saturated fat.
- Food marketing: Unhealthy foods are widely and aggressively marketed to kids, particularly youth of color. Companies use tactics like licensed characters to appeal to kids, and strategies like specialized product design, language and cultural references, cause-related marketing, and personalized digital advertisements to target

youth of color. Food marketing increases kids' desire for, purchases of, and intake of unhealthy foods.

- Food labeling: The high prevalence of nutrition claims in the U.S. packaged food supply makes it difficult for consumers to tell when a product is unhealthy. For example, claims like ''Natural'' on sugary fruit drinks mislead parents into thinking that drinks don't contain added sugar when they do. Although recent updates to the Nutrition Facts Panel, like requiring information about added sugar, are applaudable, most consumers do not always use the information and it is hard to understand for consumers with low education levels.
- Food pricing: Sugary drinks and ultraprocessed foods tend to be cheaper than minimally processed or whole foods. Parents report wanting to buy healthy foods but being unable to afford to.
- Retail environment: Sugary drinks and ultraprocessed foods are ubiquitous in food stores and are often placed in the checkout, end caps, and at locations and heights that kids are more likely to see and pester their parents to get.
- School foods: The Healthy Hunger-Free Kids Act improved school nutrition. However, most of the calories kids consume at schools still come from ultraprocessed foods, and unhealthy food marketing in schools is very common.
- Industry interference: The food industry has funded professional societies and research scientists to change the narrative on what causes obesity and type 2 diabetes, preventing policy progress.

What policies are needed based on global evidence.

- Front-of-package labels: Front-of-package nutrition labels that are clear, grab attention, and are easy to understand can help consumers make informed, healthier choices. In 2016, Chile was the first of now 10 countries to implement mandatory front-of-package nutrient warnings on unhealthy foods. The policy incentivized the food industry to cut sugar, sodium, and saturated fat in the food supply with no adverse impact on wages or employment. The policy also reduced unhealthy food purchases. The FDA is currently researching front-of-package labels and should consider a design like Chile's, which has been demonstrated in U.S. experimental research to outperform other label types.

- Food marketing restrictions: Voluntary corporate initiatives to restrict marketing are ineffective. Mandatory restrictions on unhealthy food marketing to children—for example, by limiting where ads appear or by reducing the use of techniques like cartoons—would help children develop preferences for healthy foods. In Chile, strong food marketing restrictions cut children's exposure to unhealthy food advertisements by 73 percent.

An additional policy is the removal of tax deductions on companies' advertising expenditures, which would make it more expensive to advertise unhealthy foods to children, cut kids' exposure, and also generate tax revenue for the government.

- Taxes: Global evidence from 50+ countries shows that sugary drink and ultraprocessed food taxes incentivize reformulation and reduce consumption. Revenue from taxes can be used to fund public health programs to further type 2 diabetes prevention, such as for fruit and vegetable subsidies for low-income families.
- Healthier school food environments: Schools should be free from the marketing, promotion, and sales of sugary drinks and ultraprocessed foods. Global evidence shows that restricting the marketing, promotion, and sales of unhealthy foods in schools reduces their availability and improves children's diets.
- Increase funding for nutrition research: With only 1.3 percent of the NIH budget, more funding for nutrition science is needed to improve diets and prevent obesity, type 2 diabetes, and other diet-related chronic diseases.

The CHAIR. Thank you very much. Our next witness is Dr. Kasia Lipska, Associate Professor of Medicine at the Yale School of Medicine, and we thank her very much for being with us.

## Statement of Kasia Lipska, M.D., M.H.S, Associate Professor of Medicine, Yale School of Medicine, New Haven, CT

Dr. LIPSKA. Thank you. Chairman Sanders and Ranking Member Cassidy, I am Dr. Kasia Lipska, Physician Scientist at the Yale School of Medicine. Thank you for the opportunity to present my testimony.

As a clinician, I take care of patients who have—who already have developed diabetes. There are now over 35 million people with type 2 diabetes in our Country. Nearly one in every third older adults has diabetes.

My focus with patients is to reduce the risk of complications of diabetes, such as heart attacks, strokes, amputations, kidney failure, and blindness. One of the biggest challenges in my clinical practice, including this past year, is still figuring out how to get my patients access to affordable treatment.

Even the best medications cannot help patients if they cannot afford them. According to a national survey, in 2021, 16 and a half percent of people with diabetes rationed their insulin because of cost.

This is not just due to lack of insurance coverage. Among Medicare beneficiaries with diabetes, 1 in 10 reported skipping, delaying, or taking less medication to save money. There has been so much excitement about the new medications and type 2 diabetes and obesity.

That is because some of the medications, including semaglutide or Ozempic, really seem to work. They not only help people lose weight, but also importantly reduce the risk of complications related to diabetes and obesity. But the price tags for these new medications are simply outrageous.

Ozempic, the brand name for semaglutide approved for type 2 diabetes and marketed by Novo Nordisk, has a U.S. list price of over $900 per month. Wegovy, the brand name for the same drug approved for obesity is $1,300 per month. If Medicare were to fully cover Wegovy for all of its beneficiaries with obesity for 1 year, we as American taxpayers would end up with a $268 billion invoice.

To give you some perspective, that is 70 percent of all the money that was spent on prescription drugs in the U.S. in 2021. And could we stop at 1 year? Probably not. What we know about semaglutide, and the related medications is that they work while people take them. However, as soon as they stop, their weight comes back.

Patients are looking at a potentially lifelong treatment, and we could be facing the most expensive subscription service in the history of medicine.

What can Congress do to fix this? Ozempic is priced at roughly $100 per month in Sweden and just $80 in Australia and France.

That is 10 percent of what we are being asked to pay. One explanation is that those governments are negotiating prices directly with the pharmaceutical companies. That is not socialized medicine. That is smart negotiating. Price negotiation is critical, but I believe we must do more.

Pharmaceutical companies have absolutely no restrictions on the launch prices of their products, nor is there any evidence that these prices are reflective of research and development costs. No amount of expert negotiation can bring down drug prices years later, when the launch price is sky high to begin with.

We have to align the launch price with the drug's value, the cost to develop and manufacture the drug, and what patients can afford. This is a rational approach that is in place in many other developed countries. But I want to be clear here, medications alone cannot be the solution to the diabetes and obesity epidemics.

We need to be more farsighted and strategic than that. Neither diabetes and obesity is a moral failure or a personal choice. Just telling people to eat less, exercise more is not going to solve the problem.

Instead, we must address the upstream causes of obesity, like holding the food industry accountable, as my fellow experts have already made clear. The reality is that the drug industry is really good at pushing its solutions and its products. Drug companies are powerful, sometimes more powerful than governments.

Novo Nordisk, which is based in Denmark, now has a market value that is bigger than its host nation's GDP. So, we must remember that drugs alone can't save us. They are only part of the solution.

We can't simply prescribe our way out of this problem. And before we sign up for that never ending subscription service and spend trillions of dollars, let's be smart consumers and have the Government at the negotiating table right from the start.

In closing, the bottom line is this, we have a food industry that profits from making people sick and a drug industry that profits from treating them. We must break that cycle. Thank you.

[The prepared statement of Dr. Lipska follows:]

## Prepared Statement of Kasia Lipska

Chairman Sanders and Ranking Member Cassidy, I am Dr. Kasia Lipska, a physician scientist at the Yale School of Medicine in the Section of Endocrinology and Metabolism. Thank you for the opportunity to present my testimony. I am here in my personal capacity as an expert in endocrinology and practicing clinician, and I am not representing the Yale School of Medicine.

My research has focused on the safety and effectiveness of medications to treat type 2 diabetes. I have evaluated trends in utilization of these medications over time and examined associated health outcomes. My overarching goal has been to generate evidence that patients and doctors can use to make decisions about what treatment is best for each individual. However, I realized that in my own practice, I was often forced to make decisions with my patients about medications—not based on scientific evidence about their safety and effectiveness—but rather on what options were affordable, even if those options were far from ideal. As a result, I expanded my research to consider cost-related barriers to treatment. In 2017, we conducted a survey in our Yale Diabetes Center and showed that 1 in 4 patients with diabetes, who were prescribed insulin, rationed this medication due to cost.[1] I became involved in advocacy efforts for affordable insulin. In addition to writing editorial pieces in national media outlets such as the New York Times,[2] 2 and testifying before the House Energy & Commerce Committee on the human impact of rising insulin costs,[3] I have worked closely with T1International, an advocacy organization that does not accept any money from the pharmaceutical industry or any other entity that might influence their ability to speak out freely.

As a clinician, I take care of patients who have already developed diabetes. There are now over 38 million people with diabetes in our Country. Nearly 1 in every 3d older adults has diabetes.[4]

---

[1] Herkert D, Vijayakumar P, Luo J, et al. Cost-Related Insulin Underuse Among Patients with Diabetes. JAMA internal medicine. 2019;179(1):112–114.

[2] Lipska KJ. Break up the insulin racket. The New York Times, Opinion, February 20, 2016; Available at: *https://www.nytimes.com/2016/02/21/opinion/sunday/break-up-the-insulin-racket.html*. Accessed July 11, 2019.

[3] Lipska, KJ, Expert Witness Testimony for the House Committee on Energy & Commerce: ''Priced out of a lifesaving drug: The human impact of rising insulin costs;'' April 2d, 2019. Available at *https://energycommerce.house.gov/sites/democrats.energycommerce.house.gov/files/documents/Testimony—Lipska—Insulin* percent20Prices.pdf Accessed June 29, 2021.

[4] Centers for Disease Control and Prevention, National Diabetes Statistics Report. Available at: *https://www.cdc.gov/diabetes/data/statistics-report/*. Accessed on December 10, 2023.

My focus with patients is to reduce the risk of complications of diabetes, such as heart attacks, strokes, amputations, kidney failure, and blindness. My clinic is in the Yale Diabetes Center in New Haven, CT where we serve over 3,000 patients with both type 1 and type 2 diabetes. About a third of our patients are insured by Medicaid, a third by Medicare, and a third have commercial insurance. New Haven's age, education, and race/ethnicity demographics reflect those of our Nation.[5] One of the biggest challenges in my clinical practice—including this past year—is still figuring out how to get my patients access to affordable treatment. This is what it's like in my clinic. I saw a 71-year-old man who is a retired auto body mechanic for follow-up the other day. He has type 2 diabetes, obesity, fatty liver disease, and coronary heart disease. He was taking metformin for his diabetes, but his blood sugars were uncontrolled. I prescribed Ozempic (semaglutide) but he was not able to fill this due to cost. We tried the other medications in the same class, but those were also expensive. I switched to Jardiance (empagliflozin), a pill for type 2 diabetes that reduces the risk of cardiovascular complications, but he had to stop this as well because our 340B program no longer offers it at a discount. He ended up on glipizide, probably the worst possible choice for his type 2 diabetes. Glipizide is associated with a risk of low blood sugar reactions and tends to result in weight gain.

Even the best medications cannot help patients if they cannot afford them. According to a national survey, in 2021, 16.5 percent of people with diabetes rationed their insulin because of cost.[6] This is not just due to lack of insurance coverage. Among Medicare beneficiaries with diabetes, 1 in 10 reported skipping, delaying, or taking less medication to save money.[7] What's more, when patients fill their perscriptions and purchase the insulin that they need, this is often extremely costly for them. Using nationally representative data from 2017 and 2018, we found that 14.1 percent of Americans reached

---

[5] 'Normal America' Is Not A Small Town of White People. April 28, 2016 available at: *https://fivethirtyeight.com/features/normal-america-is-not-a-small-town-of-white-people/*. "The metropolitan area that looks most like the U.S. is New Haven, Connecticut" based on age, educational attainment, race, and ethnicity metrics.

[6] Gaffney A, Himmelstein DU, Woolhandler S. Prevalence and Correlates of Patient Rationing of Insulin in the United States: A National Survey. Annals of internal medicine. 2022;175(11):1623–1626.

[7] Assistant Secretary for Planning and Evaluation (ASPE) Report, "Prescription Drug Affordability among Medicare Beneficiaries", January 19, 2022, available at: *https://aspe.hhs.gov/sites/default/files/documents/1e2879846aa54939c56efeec9c6f96f0/prescription-drug-afford- ability.pdf*. Accessed on December 10, 2023.

catastrophic levels of out-of-pocket spending on insulin, defined as spending more than 40 percent of their disposable family income on insulin alone.[8]

There has been progress in making insulin affordable—in large part due to tireless advocacy efforts by many people living with the disease, including organizations like T1International, fighting for access to insulin for all. And progress has been made thanks to the many policies that you have proposed or passed into law to improve insulin affordability. But on the whole, insulin is still way too expensive. My patients continue to struggle to pay for this drug. Over a century ago, inventors of insulin gave their patent to the University of Toronto, for $1, so that humankind would have affordable access to the drug forever.[9] Instead, drug companies have been very resourceful at controlling the market, gaming the patent system to block more affordable competitors, inflating their product prices ever since. And now that there are many new medications for diabetes, we must apply the lessons we learned from insulin to not make the same mistakes again.

There has been so much excitement about the new medications in type 2 diabetes and obesity. That's because some of the medications, including semaglutide (marketed by Novo Nordisk as Ozempic for type 2 diabetes and as Wegovy for obesity), really seem to work. They not only help people lose weight but also reduce the risk of complications related to diabetes and obesity.[10,11] In recent trials, these medications reduced the risk of cardiovascular complications by 20–25 percent.[10,11]

But the price tags for these new medications are outrageous. Ozempic, the brand name for semaglutide approved for type 2 diabetes, has a U.S. list price of over $900 per month. Wegovy, the brand name for the same drug approved for obesity, is $1,300 per month.[12] If Medicare were to fully cover Wegovy for all of its beneficiaries with obesity, we as American taxpayers would end up with a $268 billion invoice.[12] To give you some perspective, that's 70 percent of all the money that was spent on prescription drugs in the U.S. in

---

[8] Bakkila BF, Basu S, Lipska KJ. Catastrophic Spending On Insulin In The United States, 2017–18. Health affairs (Project Hope). 2022;41(7):1053–1060.

[9] Bliss M. The discovery of insulin. Chicago: University of Chicago Press, 2013.

[10] Marso SP, Bain SC, Consoli A, et al. Semaglutide and Cardiovascular Outcomes in Patients with Type 2 Diabetes. N Engl J Med. 2016.

[11] Lincoff AM, Brown-Frandsen K, Colhoun HM, et al. Semaglutide and Cardiovascular Outcomes in Obesity without Diabetes. N Engl J Med. 2023.

[12] Baig K, Dusetzina SB, Kim DD, Leech AA. Medicare Part D Coverage of Antiobesity Medications—Challenges and Uncertainty Ahead. N Engl J Med. 2023;388(11):961–963.

2021.[13] And could we stop at 1 year? Probably not. What we know about semaglutide, and the related medications, is that they work while people take them. However, as soon as they stop, their weight comes back.[14] So patients are looking at a potentially lifelong treatment and we could be facing the most expensive subscription service in the history of medicine.

How do we find a way to make these drugs affordable? We can't assume that this will simply get better with time, as patents expire after several years. There is just too much money on the table and the pharmaceutical industry is not about to walk away.

What can Congress do to help patients like mine? Ozempic is priced at roughly $100 per month in Sweden and just $80 in Australia and France.[15] That's 10 percent of what we are being asked to pay. One explanation is that those governments are negotiating prices directly with the pharmaceutical companies.[16] That's not socialized medicine. That's smart negotiating. That's a group of people leveraging their buying power to get a good deal.

The Inflation Reduction Act already authorizes the Secretary of the Department of Health and Human Services (HHS) to negotiate prices with pharmaceutical companies under specific provisions, and for a limited set of drugs. Notably, 4 out of the 10 initial medications selected for negotiation are medications for type 2 diabetes. But neither semaglutide nor the related medications in the same class are currently on the list of these drugs. As a result, millions of Americans are being asked to pay an impossible price—almost $900 a month—to get treatment that has the potential to change their lives. Many simply can't. That money is needed to pay rent, buy groceries, or make a car payment. So they go without. I see these patients every week in my clinic.

Price negotiation is critical, but I believe we must do more. Pharmaceutical companies have absolutely no restrictions on the ''launch prices'' of their products, nor is there any evidence that these prices are

---

[13] Centers for Medicare & Medicaid Services, National Health Expenditure Accounts, National Health Expenditures 2021 Highlights, available at: *https://www.cms.gov/files/document/highlights.pdf.* Accessed on December 10, 2023.

[14] Wilding JPH, Batterham RL, Davies M, et al. Weight regain and cardiometabolic effects after withdrawal of semaglutide: The STEP 1 trial extension. Diabetes Obes Metab. 2022;24(8):1553–1564.

[15] Peterson Center on Healthcare-Kaiser Family Foundation, ''How do prices of drugs for weight loss in the U.S. compare to peer nations' prices?'' Available at: *https:/www.healthsystemtracker.org/brief/prices-of-drugs-for-weight-loss-in-the-us-and-peer-nations/* Accessed on December 10, 2023.

[16] Vokinger KN, Naci H. Negotiating Drug Prices in the U.S.-Lessons from Europe. JAMA Health Forum. 2022;3(12):e224801.

reflective of research and development costs.[17] No amount of expert negotiation can bring down drug prices years later when the launch price is anchored to be sky-high. We have to align the launch price with the drug's value, the costs to develop and manufacture the drug, and what patients can afford. This is a rational approach that is in place in many other developed countries.

But I want to be clear here: medications alone cannot be the solution to the diabetes and obesity epidemics. We need to be more far sighted and strategic than that. Neither diabetes nor obesity is a moral failure or a personal choice. Just telling people to eat less and exercise more is not going to solve the problem—that strategy has failed thus far. Instead, we must address the upstream causes of obesity on the systemic level, such as reducing food deserts and improving built environments.[18] (As my fellow experts have already made clear.)

The reality is that the drug industry is really good at pushing its solutions and its products. Drug companies are powerful, sometimes more powerful than governments. Novo Nordisk, which is based in Denmark, now has a market value that is bigger than its host nation's GDP.[19] And so, perhaps inevitably, the path of least resistance will be for us to prescribe our way out of this problem. So I leave with you two thoughts:

1. drugs alone can't save us, they're only part of the solution; and
2. before we sign up for that never-ending ''subscription service,'' and spend trillions of dollars, let's be smart consumers and have the government at the negotiating table, right from the start. Every extra dollar spent on these exorbitantly priced drugs is another dollar not available to address the systemic issues contributing to diabetes and obesity in the first place.

---

[17] Wouters OJ, Berenbrok LA, He M, Li Y, Hernandez I. Association of Research and Development Investments with Treatment Costs for New Drugs Approved From 2009 to 2018. JAMA network open. 2022;5(9):e2218623.

[18] Vandevijvere S, De Pauw R, Djojosoeparto S, et al. Upstream Determinants of Overweight and Obesity in Europe. Curr Obes Rep. 2023.

[19] Bloomberg News, ''Novo's Value Surpasses Denmark GDP After Obesity Drug Boost'', available at: *https://www.bloomberg.com/news/articles/2023—08—09/wegovy-pushes-novo-nordisk-nvo-market-value-above-denmark-gdp*. Accessed on December 10, 2023.

## Summary Statement of Kasia Lipska

*Even the best medications cannot help patients if they cannot afford them.* According to a national survey, in 2021, 16.5 percent of people with diabetes rationed their insulin because of cost. This is not just due to lack of insurance coverage. Among Medicare beneficiaries with diabetes, 1 in 10 reported skipping, delaying, or taking less medication to save money.

There has been so much excitement about the new medications in type *2 diabetes and obesity*. That's because some of the medications, including semaglutide, really seem to work. They not only help people lose weight but also reduce the risk of complications related to diabetes and obesity.

*But the price tags for these new medications are outrageous.* Ozempic, the brand name for semaglutide approved for type 2 diabetes, has a U.S. list price of over $900 per month. Wegovy, the brand name for the same drug approved for obesity is $1,300 per month. If Medicare were to fully cover Wegovy for all of its beneficiaries with obesity, we as American taxpayers would end up with a $268 billion invoice. To give you some perspective, that's 70 percent of all the money that was spent on prescription drugs in the U.S. in 2021. And could we stop at 1 year? Probably not. What we know about semaglutide, and the related medications, is that they work while people take them. However, as soon as they stop, their weight comes back. So we could be looking at lifelong treatment here and then we're potentially talking about the most expensive subscription service in the history of medicine.

*How do we find a way to make these drugs affordable?* Ozempic is priced at roughly $100 per month in Sweden and just $80 in Australia and France. That's 10 percent of what we are being asked to pay. One explanation is that those governments are negotiating prices directly with the pharmaceutical companies. That's not socialized medicine. That's smart negotiating. That's a group of people leveraging their buying power to get a good deal.

Price negotiation is critical, but I believe we must do more. Pharmaceutical companies have absolutely no restrictions on the "launch prices" of their products. No amount of expert negotiation can bring down drug prices when the launch price is sky-high. *We have to align the launch price with the drug's value, the costs to develop and manufacture the drug, and what patients can afford.* This is a rational approach that is in place in many other developed countries.

But I want to be clear here: *medications alone cannot be the solution* to the diabetes and obesity twin epidemics. We need to be more far sighted and strategic than that. Neither diabetes nor obesity is a moral failure or a personal choice. Just telling people to eat less and exercise more is not going to solve the problem—that strategy has failed thus far. Instead, *we must address the upstream causes of obesity on the systemic level,* such as reducing food deserts and improving built environments.

The reality is that the drug industry is really good at pushing its solutions and its products. And so, perhaps inevitably, the path of least resistance will be for us to prescribe our way out of this problem. So I leave with you two thoughts: [1] drugs alone can't save us, they're only part of the solution; and [2] before we sign up for that never-ending ''subscription service,'' and spend trillions of dollars, let's be smart consumers and have the government at the negotiating table, right from the start. *Every extra dollar spent on these exorbitantly priced drugs is another dollar not available to address the systemic issues contributing to diabetes and obesity in the first place.*

The CHAIR. Thank you very much.

Senator Cassidy, want to introduce your witnesses?

Senator CASSIDY. Yes, thank you, Mr. Chairman. Pleased to first introduce Mrs. Natalie Stanback, a mother to a type 1 diabetes patient. Mrs. Stanback provides an insightful, personal perspective on the issues of children with type 1 diabetes and their parents' encounter.

In 2015, Mrs. Stanback's daughter Nadia was diagnosed with type 1 diabetes, and apparently her family has a strong family history of type 1 diabetes, unrelated to obesity. Natalie volunteers with JDRF, the Juvenile Diabetes Research Foundation, to advocate for type 1 diabetes research. Earlier this year, she served as chair of the JDRF's children's Congress.

She lives in Texas with her husband and three kids. Thank you for joining us. I look forward to your testimony.

## Statement of Natalie Stanback, Volunteer, JDRF, Lewisville, TX

Mrs. STANBACK. Chairman Sanders, Ranking Member Dr. Cassidy, Members of the Committee, thank you for inviting me to testify today. I am here because unfortunately, I am deeply familiar with the many challenges presented by type 1 diabetes, or T1D.

I do not have this disease, but my 11 year old daughter Nadia does, and she lives with it. My brother died from complications of T1D when he was only 38 years old, so you can imagine the fear that I felt when Nadia was diagnosed at the age of three. It was overwhelming, to say the least.

Nadia does not know life without diabetes. We are blessed to have access to the best medical care, which helps her live the life she wants to live. She has an insulin pump and a continuous glucose monitor. She plays soccer and runs track. She looks like a normal kid, and in most ways she is.

But diabetes is always there, 365 days a year, 24/7. This disease is hard, and it is cumbersome. We are an emotionally positive family, glass half full, but this disease is still hard on all of us, but especially it is hard on Nadia. She can't eat without calculating how many carbohydrates are in the food so that she can dose the correct amount of insulin.

Her blood sugar levels can go low during soccer games, which forces her to sit out, and then treat it, and then get back in the game if there is still time. She has to deal with the needles necessary to change insulin pump infusionsites and glucose monitoring sensors in a way that many adults would and still do struggle with.

Then prescriptions and doctor's appointments must be diligently managed. My daughter is brave. She is responsible and she is miraculous, but it is still so very hard every day, not just for her, but for all those around her.

Her siblings, extended family members, teachers, coaches, friends, friends' parents, everyone needs to understand Nadia's needs and how they can help, especially in the case of an emergency. It takes a village to raise a child. It takes a city to raise a child with diabetes. I know that the Members of this Committee are aware of the realities of diabetes and have championed this cause for years.

I am grateful. I was honored to chair JDRF's children's Congress this past summer, and I know the amazing delegates and guardians you all met are so grateful too. Having you as champions has helped us get to where we are today.

In fact, SPD supported research directly contributed to the development of the incredible devices that Nadia relies on every day. They could still be—they could still be years in the future, if not for the support of the SPD.

What my daughter and what every parent of a child with diabetes needs, and what every person affected with diabetes needs is a cure. Something that removes the thousands of medical decisions we must make every day so that we can focus on everything else in life.

For my daughter, that would mean focusing on scoring goals on the soccer field and doing well in school, not whether she will go dangerously low or high in blood sugar in the process. Research can make that happen.

The STP has been foundational to nearly every advance in pursuit of that ultimate goal, which is cures. I am excited about the progress in therapies to delay T1D onset and those at risk of developing the disease.

Anyone who is able to take advantage of delaying T1D onset is receiving an incredible gift, time without T1D. I wish that Nadia could have had that opportunity. I do believe that someday Nadia will receive that ultimate gift, life without T1D. We have made incredible progress toward curing T1D through cell therapies.

This research is happening right now. I do not know when she will receive that gift. No one does. But I do know the best way to bring that day closer is long term, sustained funding for the special diabetes program. This research must continue. As a mom, I do not want my daughter to face a lifetime with diabetes.

With STP funded research, I no cures are possible. I know a life free of insulin pumps and monitors and the looming threat of complications is on the horizon, but only if the brilliant minds who have gotten us this far have the resources they need to get us across that finish line. And until then, we need affordable insulin.

The Insulin Act would help us make that more of a reality, so I urge you for your support. Thank you so very much for your time, and I look forward to your questions.

[The prepared statement of Mrs. Stanback follows:]

## Prepared Statement of Natalie Stanback

Chairman Sanders, Ranking Member Dr. Cassidy, Members of the Committee— thank you for inviting me to testify today. I'm here because, unfortunately, I'm deeply familiar with the many challenges presented by type 1 diabetes—T1D. I don't have this disease, but my eleven-year-old daughter, Nadia, lives with it.

My brother died from complications from T1D when he was only 24 years old so you can imagine the fear I felt when Nadia was diagnosed at the age of 3. It was overwhelming.

Nadia doesn't know life without diabetes. We are blessed to have access to the best medical care, which helps her live the life she wants to live. She has an insulin pump and a continuous glucose monitor. She plays soccer and runs track. She looks like a normal kid, and, in most ways, she is.

But diabetes is always there 365 days a year 24/7. This disease is hard. We're a very emotionally positive family—definitely glass half full. But this disease is hard. On all of us, but especially Natalie. She can't eat without calculating how many carbohydrates are in the food to dose the correct amount of insulin. Her blood sugar level can get low during soccer games, which forces her to sit out, treat it, and then get back in the game if there's still time. She has to deal with the needles necessary to change insulin pump infusionsites and glucose monitoring sensors in a way many adults would struggle with. And prescriptions and doctor appointments must be diligently managed.

My daughter is brave, responsible—she is miraculous. But it is still so very hard, every day. And not just for her, but for all those around her.

Her siblings, extended family members, teachers, coaches, friends, friends' parents—everyone needs to understand Nadia's needs and how they can help, especially in case of an emergency.

If it takes a village to raise a child, it takes a city to raise a child with diabetes.

I know that the Members of this Committee are aware of the realities of diabetes and have championed this cause for years. I am grateful. I was honored to chair JDRF's Children's Congress this past summer and I know the amazing delegates and guardians you met are grateful, too.

Having you as champions has helped us get to where we are today. In fact, SPD- supported research directly contributed to the development of the incredible devices that Nadia relies on every day. They could still be years in the future if not for the support of the SDP.

What my daughter, what every parent of a child with diabetes needs, and every person affected by diabetes needs is a cure. Something that removes the thousands of medical decisions we must make every day so that we can focus on everything else in life. For my daughter, that would mean focusing on scoring goals on the soccer field and doing well in school, not whether she will get dangerously low or high blood sugar in the process.

Research can make that happen. The SDP has been foundational to nearly every advance in pursuit of that ultimate goal: cures.

I am excited about the progress in therapies to delay T1D onset in those at risk of developing the disease. Anyone who is able to take advantage of delaying T1D onset is receiving an incredible gift—time without T1D. I wish that Nadia could have had that opportunity.

I do believe that, someday, Nadia will receive the ultimate gift—life without T1D. We have made incredible progress toward curing T1D through cell therapies. This research is happening right now. I don't know when she will get that gift—no one does—but I do know the best way to bring that day closer is long-term, sustained funding of the Special Diabetes Program. This research must continue.

As a mom, I don't want my daughter to face a lifetime with diabetes. With SDP- funded research, I know cures are possible. I know a life free of insulin pumps and monitors and the looming threat of complications is on the horizon—but only if the brilliant minds who have gotten us this far have the resources, they need to get us across the finish line.

Until then, we need affordable insulin. The INSULIN Act would help make that more of a reality. I urge your support.

Thank you very much for your time and I look forward to your questions.

## Summary Statement of Natalie Stanback

Chairman Sanders, Ranking Member Dr. Cassidy, Members of the Committee— thank you for inviting me to testify today. I am here because, unfortunately, I am deeply familiar with the many challenges presented by type 1 diabetes—T1D. I do not have this disease, but my eleven-year-old daughter, Nadia, lives with it.

My brother died from complications from T1D when he was only 24 years old so you can imagine the fear I felt when Nadia was diagnosed at the age of 3. It was overwhelming.

Nadia does not know life without diabetes. We are blessed to have access to the best medical care, which helps her live the life she wants to live. She has an insulin pump and a continuous glucose monitor. She plays soccer and runs track. She looks like a normal kid, and, in most ways, she is.

But diabetes is always there 365 days a year 24/7. This disease is hard.

My daughter is brave, responsible—she is miraculous. But it is still so extremely hard, every day. And not just for her, but for all those around her. Her siblings, extended family members, teachers, coaches, friends, friends' parents—everyone needs to understand Nadia's needs and how they can help, especially in case of an emergency. If it takes a village to raise a child, it takes a city to raise a child with diabetes. I know that the Members of this Committee are aware of the realities of diabetes and have championed this cause for years. I am grateful. I was honored to chair JDRF's Children's Congress this past summer and I know the amazing delegates and guardians you met are grateful, too.

Having you as champions has helped us get to where we are today. In fact, SPD- supported research directly contributed to the development of the incredible devices the SDP.

What my daughter, what every parent of a child with diabetes needs, and every person affected by diabetes needs is a cure. Something that removes the thousands of medical decisions we must make every day so that we can focus on everything else in life. For my daughter, which would mean focusing on scoring goals on the soccer field and doing well in school, not whether she will get dangerously low or high blood sugar in the process.

Research can make that happen.

As a mom, I do not want my daughter to face a lifetime with diabetes. With SDP- funded research, I know cures are possible. I know a life free of insulin pumps and monitors and the looming threat of complications is on the horizon—but only if the brilliant minds who have gotten us this far have the resources, they need to get us across the finish line.

Until then, we need affordable insulin. The INSULIN Act would help make that more of a reality. I urge your support.

Thank you very much for your time and I look forward to your questions.

Senator CASSIDY. And now I have the privilege of introducing the next witness, Dr. Aaron Kowalski, the Chief Executive Officer and President of JDRF. In his role as CEO and President of JDRF, Dr. Kowalski is responsible for advancing and funding type 1 diabetes research by working closely with academics and the type 1 diabetes community.

He is also a scientist, and I am told, and this is apparently not HIPPA protected, you also have type 1 diabetes. I always got to throw that in there, Dr. Kowalski, and make sure I don't get busted.

Dr. Kowalski has authored a number of type 1 diabetes research articles focusing upon diabetes standards of care and the artificial pancreas. He has a doctorate in microbiology and molecular genetics from Rutgers. I look forward to your testimony, sir. Thank you for joining us.

## Statement of Aaron J. Kowalski, PhD., Chief Executive Officer, JDRF, New York, NY

Dr. KOWALSKI. Thank you. Chairman Sanders, Ranking Member Dr. Cassidy, Members of the Committee, thank you so much for inviting me to testify and your interest in diabetes. I am Dr. Aaron Kowalski, CEO of JDRF, the leading global not for profit focused on type 1 diabetes.

As a scientist by training, and Dr. Cassidy, as a person living with type 1 diabetes, I am honored to work for JDRF for the past 19 years, 4 of which in my current role. I would like to start with a thank you.

Because of your incredible bipartisan support and leadership, and the steadfast leadership of the Senate Diabetes Caucus Co- Chair Senator Collins, who just had to leave, unfortunately, and Senator Shaheen, the Special Diabetes Program, the STP, and the Special Diabetes Program for Indians, the STPI, are making a tremendous difference in the lives of people with diabetes and for their, our hope for the future.

These programs have helped fundamentally change what it means to live with type 1 diabetes and have put new life changing therapies in our hands and have brought us closer to cures.

JDRF and our countless volunteers are so grateful for the Committee—that the Committee recognizes the importance of building on this progress with the approval of S. 1855, the Special Diabetes Program Reauthorization Act.

We thank you, and we continue to work with your colleagues to ensure the 2-year $170 million per year for each program is enacted. Let me highlight for you a few of the many exciting breakthroughs that have resulted in the investment in the STP that gives us so much hope for a brighter future.

Because of STP funding, we have a new therapy approved, the first ever what we would call disease modifying therapy, it is called Tzield, that delays the onset of type 1 diabetes and the need for insulin for nearly 3 years.

This is a landmark, first time in 100 years we have ever changed the course of type 1. Other such therapies are advancing in the research pipeline. This is huge progress. Delaying the onset has a tremendous impact on the daily lives of people at risk for type 1, their families, and the overall health care system.

To take full advantage of Tzield and therapies on the horizon, we need to ensure widespread screening for the risk factors that trigger type 1. In June, the FDA approved the first ever cell therapy for adults with type 1, those who are unable to maintain average blood glucose levels due to severe episodes of hypoglycemia.

This therapy will allow some patients to live without external insulin for several years. This therapy could also have promise for the estimated 8 million people T2D, type 2, who also rely on insulin administration every single day. This would not have happened without STP funding.

Another game changer for people with diabetes is technology to better manage blood sugar levels. I and many others with type 1 wear an artificial pancreas system or AP systems. It consists of an insulin pump, a continuous glucose monitor, and a computer program called an algorithm that allows the pump and the CGM to communicate with each other and give the right amount of insulin at the right time.

AP systems aren't perfect. They don't replace what you lost when you developed type 1 diabetes, but they do make life better. Better blood sugar control and easier diabetes management. Several systems are on the market now and next gen systems are in the research pipeline.

Individuals with type 2 are also benefiting from these technologies. Many now use CGM to gain valuable information about how their food, exercise, stress, and other factors impact their lives, and help them better manage their blood sugar levels to improve their health. Just this last week, the ADA standards of care were updated to reflect the importance of diabetes devices and recommended them to patients right away when they are diagnosed.

Continued support of the STP will enable several long term T1D oriented research programs and clinical trial networks to continue their important work. It will enable researchers to explore new opportunities.

For example, highly beneficial SGLT inhibitors, drugs that lower blood sugar by preventing kidneys from re-absorbing glucose are approved type 2, but not for people with type 1.

We need to develop strategies to ensure these drugs can be safely used by type 1 people, which could reduce the costly and devastating impact of heart and kidney disease. Research for both type 1 and type 2 is critical to gain further understanding, advanced therapies, find cures, and JDRF and others are significantly investing in this research.

But absent Government support and investment, these advancements will slow. The cost of diabetes will rise. We need Congress to move swiftly and enact the STP and STPI funding contained in S. 1855.

Until cures, we need affordable insulin for all those who need it to live. JDRF supports the bipartisan Insulin Act of 2023, led by Senators Collins and Shaheen, and calls on Congress to support its enactment.

Thank you again for this opportunity to testify and I look forward to your questions.

[The prepared statement of Dr. Kowalski follows:]

## Prepared Statement of Aaron J. Kowalski

Chairman Sanders, Ranking Member Dr. Cassidy, and Members of the Committee, I am Dr. Aaron J. Kowalski, Chief Executive Officer for JDRF, the leading global organization harnessing the power of research, advocacy, and community engagement to advance life-changing breakthroughs for type 1 diabetes—T1D. As a scientist by training, a person living with T1D, and someone with a brother with T1D, I have been honored to work for JDRF and to represent individuals and families impacted by T1D for the past 19 years, four of which have been in my current role.

I am also honored to testify and appreciate the Committee's focus on diabetes. I would like to start with a thank you. Because of your bipartisan leadership and support, and the steadfast leadership of Senate Diabetes Caucus Co-Chairs, Senators Susan Collins and Jeanne Shaheen, the Special Diabetes Program and the Special Diabetes Program for Indians (SDPI) are making a tremendous difference in the lives of people with diabetes and their hope for the future. These programs have helped to fundamentally change what it means to live with diabetes, have put new life-changing therapies in our hands, and have brought us closer to cures.

JDRF and our countless volunteers are grateful the Committee recognizes the importance of maintaining this momentum and building upon this progress with the approval of S. 1855, the Special Diabetes Program Reauthorization Act of 2023. We thank you and continue to work with your colleagues to ensure the 2-year, $170 million per year for each program, is enacted.

## Diabetes—A Costly and Burdensome Disease

Far too many people are aware of ''diabetes'' but do not know the difference between type 1 diabetes (T1D) and type 2 diabetes (T2D). T1D is an autoimmune disease in which a person's pancreas stops producing insulin, a hormone that enables a person to utilize energy from food. The condition lasts a lifetime, and people with T1D must take insulin to live. T2D is a metabolic disease. With T2D, the body still produces insulin but cannot use it effectively.

Today, more than 37 million Americans have diabetes and 96 million have prediabetes.[20] Of those with diabetes, JDRF estimates that 1.4 million people have T1D. Diabetes affects people of all ages and races across the country. The complications that result from the condition are significant—ranging from heart disease and strokes to lower-limb amputations—and reduce life expectancy by at least 10 years in people with diabetes compared to people without diabetes. As a result of the breadth and impact, the total annual cost for diabetes in 2022 was $412.9B, including $306.6B in direct medical costs and $106.3B in indirect costs.[21]

Research for both T1D and T2D is critical to gain further understanding, advance therapies, and find cures for both conditions. JDRF and others are investing significantly in research, but absent additional investments the advances will slow significantly, while the costs of diabetes continue to rise exponentially.

## JDRF—Partnering with the Federal Government

Before I share some of the exciting breakthroughs resulting from the SDP, I want Congress to know that JDRF's private funding works hand in hand with SDP funding to ensure that the most important and promising research projects have the support they need. JDRF accelerates the path to cures by raising funds and allocating them to T1D research and therapy development, as well as by leveraging our expertise and leadership to bring in additional funding and supporters.

I am proud to say that JDRF has invested more than $2.5 billion in research funding since our founding in 1970. And through direct research investments and partnerships within the public and private sectors, including through the SDP, we helped raise $473 million for T1D research and therapy development in JDRF's 2022 fiscal year. Investments from the JDRF T1D Fund, which is a separate mission-driven venture philanthropy fund focused on equity investments in companies developing life-changing T1D products,

---

[20] Centers for Disease Control and Prevention. National Diabetes Statistics Report website. *https://www.cdc.gov/diabetes/data/statistics-report/index.html*. Accessed July 6, 2023.

[21] American Diabetes Association. New American Diabetes Association Report Finds Annual Costs of Diabetes to be $412.9 Billion. *https://diabetes.org/newsroom/press-releases/new-american-diabetes-association-report-finds-annual-costs-diabetes-be* (2023).

is a part of this total. This partnership between the public and private sectors is what it takes to deliver major advances for T1D research.

## The Special Diabetes Program—Accelerating Breakthroughs

There has been tremendous progress that gives us hope for a brighter future. Here are some examples of the advancements that are exciting to the T1D community where the SDP played a role.

## First Disease-Modifying Therapy Brought to Market

The SDP enabled the creation of TrialNet, the largest clinical network for T1D. TrialNet conducted the clinical trials that led to the November 2022 U.S. Food and Drug Administration (FDA) approval of Tzield, the first disease-modifying therapy for individuals at-risk for developing T1D. This therapy can delay T1D onset for almost 3 years; other therapies to delay and prevent onset are advancing in the research pipeline.

A delay in the onset of T1D has a tremendous impact on the daily lives of people at risk for T1D, their families, and the overall healthcare system. It frees them from the constant burden and stress of blood glucose monitoring and insulin administration. It frees them from the worry and fear of short-and long-term complications, while giving them the opportunity to learn more about disease management. And it enables one to avoid the medical emergency that often accompanies a T1D diagnosis. This is both clinically and emotionally meaningful.

With a therapy to delayT1D onset and others on the horizon, screening for the risk factors that trigger T1D is even more important. TrialNet has a screening program for those with a direct relative who has T1D; however, anyone who tests positive for risk factors may be eligible to enroll in a clinical trial. JDRF launched T1Detect, a community-based education and awareness program to expand screening to the general population. JDRF is also studying the age or ages when screening should be done. We know the need to focus on screening is great and look forward to talking with you further about it.

## Advances in Cell Therapies

Another recent exciting development in diabetes research is the June 2023 FDA approval of the first cell therapy for adults with T1D. The approval is specifically for adults unable to maintain average blood glucose levels due to repeated severe episodes of low blood glucose levels or hypoglycemia. This therapy, with the use of immunosuppression, takes deceased donor islets and places them into people with T1D. This is an important first for the diabetes community, as it is a therapy that allows some patients to go without any injected or infused insulin for several years. This therapy could also have promise for the estimated eight million Americans with T2D who rely on insulin administration every day. Clinical trial data resulting from the SDP-supported Clinical Islet Transplantation Consortium contributed to this pivotal step toward identifying cures.

## Artificial Pancreas Systems

Yet another area of progress that is a real game changer for people with T1D is technology to better manage blood glucose levels. An artificial pancreas (AP) system consists of an insulin pump, a continuous glucose monitor (CGM), and a computer program called an algorithm that allows the pump and CGM to communicate with each other to give the right amount of insulin at the right time—much like the pancreas does in people without T1D. AP systems are not perfect, but they allow people to think about their diabetes a little less and have better blood glucose control, which improves the quality of life of those impacted by T1D and helps to mitigate costly and burdensome long-term diabetes-related complications. I was very involved in the development of AP systems and the approval process, and I'm thrilled to see the benefits that have resulted for myself, my brother who also lives with T1D, and the entire diabetes community.

SDP-funded research laid the early groundwork for developing AP systems. In fact, SDP funds contributed to the first fully automated insulin-dosing system being made available to patients in 2017, five to 7 years earlier than expected. Positive results from SDP-supported clinical trials since then have led to other FDA-approved systems and next-generation AP devices that have outperformed first-generation devices in children, adolescents, and young adults.

Individuals with T2D and athletes are also benefiting from some of this research. Many are now using CGMs to better monitor their blood glucose levels; gain valuable information about how food, exercise, stress, and other factors impact their levels; and better manage their levels for improved health or peak performance.

## The Special Diabetes Program for Indians (SDPI)—Making a Difference

The SDP's sister program, the SDPI, is also demonstrating significant progress to- ward the prevention and treatment of T2D in American Indian and Alaska Native communities, which are impacted disproportionally by the disease. The SDPI serves 780,000 American Indians and Alaska Natives across 302 programs in 35 states. The program focuses on community-directed approaches that are culturally based.

Since the beginning of the SDPI, blood glucose levels have decreased by 11 percent, average LDL cholesterol risk factors have reduced by 25 percent, diabetes-related kidney disease has been cut by more than half, fewer people are developing diabetes, and primary prevention and weight management programs for Native youth have increased. That's amazing. These successes will continue, and even greater progress will be made with the continued Federal investment contained in S. 1855.

## Future Opportunities—Building on the Momentum

While the opportunities before us are abundant, here are a few examples in need of funding with the next SDP renewal.

- Fund Long-Term Research Programs and Clinical Trials

Continued support of the SDP would keep several long-term T1D-oriented research programs and clinical trial networks running strong, enabling them to continue their work which has yielded so many exciting and promising discoveries. For example, The Environmental Determinants of Diabetes in the Young (TEDDY) study of 8,600 children, enrolled at birth and being followed until they are 15 years old, seeks to understand which environmental factors trigger or protect against T1D onset. Information on diet, infections, and other exposures is being analyzed from children who are progressing toward—or now have—full T1D onset. Results to date indicate that there are multiple pathways leading to T1D. Further investigation is needed to develop strategies to prevent the onset of the disease, ranging from a vaccine to specific dietary changes. The data collected from this study could also benefit other autoimmune diseases, such as celiac disease.

- Protect Heart and Kidney Health for Those with T1D

SGLT inhibitors, such as Invokana, Farxiga and Jardiance, protect heart and kidney health for people with type 2 diabetes but are not yet FDA approved for people with T1D. There is an immediate need to develop evidence-based strategies to ensure these drugs can be used safely by people with T1D, which could significantly reduce costly and devastating impacts of heart and kidney disease.

A recent study shows that for the current population living with T1D, lowering End Stage Renal Disease rates by 50 percent is expected to generate Medicare savings that build over time. At the 10-year mark, the cumulative savings to Medicare are $5.1 billion. By the 25-year mark, Medicare savings reach $13.6 billion.[22] These savings estimates do not incorporate individuals who will be diagnosed in the future and therefore are conservative.

- Investigate Cardiovascular Disease in People with T1D

Cardiovascular disease (CVD) in people with T1D is not as well studied as in people with T2D, even though it is a major cause of death in people with T1D. There is a major unmet need to identify the mechanisms that promote earlier development of CVD in people with T1D, to learn and develop new interventions to prevent and treat it.

## Long-term, Uninterrupted SDP Support—A Critical Need

The critical research supported by the SDP requires lengthy periods to achieve optimal results. A long-term reauthorization would allow the National Institute

[22] Winn, A, Skandari, R, O'Grady, M, and Huang, E. ''Potential Medicare Savings of Reduced End Stage Renal Disease in Patients with Diabetes,'' May 2023. Unpublished white paper.

of Diabetes and Digestive and Kidney Diseases to carefully plan the use of funds, which are directed toward new and ongoing clinical trials that take multiple years to complete.

Technology development also takes time. The noteworthy progress in developing artificial pancreas and other glucose management technologies has been spurred by long-term SDP support, as I noted earlier. For the scientists who conduct the research, long-term, sustained funding is incredibly important. With the uncertainty of sustained funding, they may pursue other research opportunities elsewhere. The assurance of long-term funding is also important to attract new talent to this field and to maintain a pipeline of future generations of scientists to conduct T1D research.

Again, I thank you Chairman Sanders, Ranking Member Dr. Cassidy, and Members of this Committee for advancing S. 1855—bipartisan legislation led by Senators Susan Collins and Jeanne Shaheen to renew the SDP and SDPI. I urge Congress to move swiftly and enact the 2-year, $170 million per year reauthorization for both programs so we can keep this exciting and life-changing momentum going.

## Insulin Affordability—Also a Critical Need

While the focus of my remarks is on the SDP and SDPI, it is important to note that people with diabetes need access to affordable insulin until we have cures. I appreciate the Committee's interest in addressing this issue, as we all know the current drug pricing system does not work for countless people who need insulin to survive. Progress has been made but we need to take the next step. JDRF urges Congress to pass the bipartisan INSULIN Act of 2023, led by Senators Susan Collins and Jeanne Shaheen, which establishes a $35 per month insulin copay cap for people with commercial insurance and includes other provisions that would make insulin more affordable for everyone, regardless of insurance status.

Thank you again for the opportunity to testify. I look forward to answering your questions.

## Summary Statement of Aaron J. Kowalski]

Thank you. Because of your bipartisan leadership and support, and the steadfast leadership of Senate Diabetes Caucus Co-Chairs, Senators Collins and Shaheen, the Special Diabetes Program—SDP—and the Special Diabetes Program for Indians— SDPI—are making a tremendous difference in the lives of people with diabetes and their hope for the future. These programs have helped to fundamentally change what it means to live with diabetes, have put new life-changing therapies in our hands, and have brought us closer to cures.

JDRF and our countless volunteers are grateful the Committee recognizes the importance of building on this progress with the approval of S. 1855, the Special Diabetes Program Reauthorization Act. We thank you and continue to work with your colleagues to ensure the 2-year, $170 million per year for each program, is enacted.

Here are a few of the many exciting breakthroughs resulting from the SDP:

A new FDA approved therapy—Tzield can delay T1D onset—and the need for insulin—for nearly 3 years. Other such therapies are in the pipeline. This has a huge impact on the lives of people at risk for T1D and the overall healthcare system. To take advantage such therapies, we must ensure widespread screening for risk factors that trigger T1D.

In June, the FDA approved the first cell therapy for adults with T1D who are unable to maintain average blood glucose levels due to severe hypoglycemia. This therapy allows some patients to live without external insulin for several years and could have promise for the estimated eight million Americans with T2D who rely on insulin administration every day.

Several artificial pancreas (AP) systems are on the market and next generation systems are in the pipeline. They're not perfect, but they typically result in better blood glucose control. Individuals with T2D are also benefiting—many now use CGMs to gain valuable information about how food, exercise, and other factors impact their levels; and better manage their blood glucose levels.

Continued SDP support will enable several long-term T1D-oriented research programs and clinical trial networks to continue their important work. And it will enable researchers to explore new opportunities. For example, highly beneficial SGLT inhibitors—drugs that lower blood sugar by preventing the kidneys from re-absorbing glucose—are approved for T2D are not yet approved for people with T1D. We need to develop strategies to ensure these drugs can safely be used by people with T1D, which could reduce the costly and devastating impacts of heart and kidney disease.

Research for both T1D and T2D is critical to gain further understanding, advance therapies, and find cures for both conditions. JDRF and others are investing significantly in research, but absent additional government investments the advances will slow significantly, while the costs of diabetes continue to rise exponentially.

We need Congress to move swiftly to enact the SDP and SDPI funding, as contained in S. 1855. And until there are cures, we need affordable insulin for all who need it to live. JDRF supports the bipartisan INSULIN Act of 2023, led by Senators Collins and Shaheen, and calls on Congress to support its enactment.

Thank you.

The CHAIR. Thank you very much, Dr. Kowalski. This familiar product is a 20 ounce bottle of Coke. Contains over 15 teaspoons of sugar, more than twice the recommended daily limit for kids under the age of 18.

This is a 12 ounce can of Coke, and according to the Center for Science in the Public Interest, people who drink one or two cans of Coke a day, ''have a 26 percent greater risk of developing type 2 diabetes than people who rarely consume such drinks. And the risks are even greater for young adults.?

Dr. Taillie, do you believe that Coca Cola and companies that make similar products should be marketing these products to children? Should there be labels on products like Coke warning people that regularly consuming sugary drinks substantially increases their chances of getting type 2 diabetes? Dr. Taillie.

Dr. TAILLIE. We know that food marketing is very effective for kids, and over 50 percent of our kids are still drinking products like Coke on a daily basis. That consumption has gone down over recent years, but still remains far too high.

These kids are being marketed products like Coke in many different ways. Increasingly, this is proliferating on social media and online, where kids aren't even able to identify it as advertising.

Kids are seeing nearly 200 ads a week for products like Coke. And so, this is really getting into their heads and creating these strong preferences for these products at a very early age.

In terms of clear labeling, we have a lot of data, both from experiments that we have done here in the U.S. and from global evidence from countries that have implemented these labels that these labels help people really clearly see when they are looking at the package that this is unhealthy.

Coke is a product that is more clear. More consumers know that sodas are unhealthy. But when we think about fruit drinks, those are the products that kids consume the most. Those are products that parents think are healthy. Those are confusing products, and they still contain a lot of sugar.

Warnings—warning labels would really help parents understand that better.

The CHAIR. Apologize for cutting you off. We don't have a lot of time. I want to go to Dr. Gearhardt.

According to your testimony, the food and beverage industry has used some of the same tactics as the tobacco industry to get our kids addicted to ultra-processed foods that are high in sugar, salt, and saturated fat.

Is that correct? Are we seeing products sold to kids similar to the style used by the tobacco companies?

Dr. GEARHARDT. Yes. So, there is documented evidence, given the intertwined histories between the tobacco industries and the processed food industries that these strategies used to sell, create market cigarettes were applied very intentionally to improve the profit margins of especially children's sugar sweetened beverages.

We know that our brains were never developed to handle this level of food reward, the amounts of sugar, how rapidly they are being delivered into the body. That these are really effective at engaging the core nerve circuitry of addiction.

The CHAIR. Thank you. Dr. Lipska, Ozempic costs about $12,000 per year in the United States, but just $2,000 here in Canada and $750 in Germany. What do these very high prices mean for your patients? Do you think your patients would be living healthier lives if we can make these drugs more affordable?

Dr. LIPSKA. Mr. Chairman, absolutely. These prices are, as I said, outrageous. And what happens is that patients cannot afford those medications and so they go without. And we know these medications have effects in terms of reducing the risk of heart disease. When people go without, they are at risk for these complications. They would be healthier if they were able to afford them.

The CHAIR. Would I be correct in saying not only do people suffer and die unnecessarily, but the cost to the health care system increases? If I can't give you a drug, you end up in the hospital. Am I correct in that?

Dr. LIPSKA. Absolutely. Absolutely correct.

The CHAIR. Okay. Senator Cassidy.

Senator CASSIDY. I am going to defer to Senator Marshall. But before I do so, I would like to have unanimous consent—Senator Collins had to leave for a just called Committee hearing. She asked that I submit for the record testimony from the Endocrine Society. I ask for unanimous consent to do so.

The CHAIR. Without objection.

[The following information can be found on page 57 in Additional Material:]

Senator CASSIDY. With that, I defer to Senator Marshall.

Senator MARSHALL. Yes. Thank you. Ranking Member and thank you, Chairman. I sit here in this Committee hearing in my head is just spinning. Been on this Committee for 3 years and I am not sure we have made any meaningful impact yet on diabetes.

A huge epidemic, as we already know this. Through these opportunities to attack the nutrition standpoint, the education standpoint, it is time to stop studying it and forming committees.

It is time to move forward with action. I think we all understand the cost of prescription drugs is part of the challenge here. It is interesting to me that in 2022, Americans spent $633 billion on prescriptions, $633 billion. Almost $500 billion of that went through the hands of our pharmacy benefit managers.

$5 out of $6 that Americans spend on prescription drugs go through the hands of pharmacy benefit managers. And of course, there is kickbacks. They give some of that money back to Medicare and insurance providers, and we have no idea who and how much those are going to.

But in case you are feeling sorry for the PBMs, they had a profits of $27 billion in 2022. $27 billion was their profit margin. Three PBMs are now ranked 4, 5, and 12 on the Fortune 500 list. So, as I look to solving this problem of prescription drugs to treat diabetes, I tried to figure out where is the biggest bang for the buck without destroying innovation.

I keep coming back to these pharmacy benefit managers. We have done incredible work so far to address this problem, but our work is not finished. We have sponsored the Drug Act, which is a bipartisan, bicameral legislation that would delink administrative fees paid to PBMs from the price of prescription drugs.

Rather than paying a percentage of the drug, that there would be a flat fee. Obviously, the PBMs are motivated to the higher the drug costs, the more they are going to benefit when they get a percentage of that. We have had great colleagues here with Senators Kaine and Braun, and we withdrew our amendment because it didn't have a CBO score at the time.

But this remains my top priority. We had the CBO estimate. Guess what? This is going to save the Federal deficit by $654 million if it is fitted into the PBM Reform Act. Senator Collins said this legislation is literally right on the money, and certainly Senator Collins has been my mentor in trying to figure out what to do with diabetes here in many ways.

The underlying issue is that PBMs favor higher priced brand insulin over insulin biosimilars. We had hoped the biosimilars coming to market would help drive this down, but it remains a challenge.

This legislation eliminates the perverse incentives of PBMs to block access to affordable insulin, biosimilars, and generic drugs. Is there anybody on the panel that would disagree that by limit—by delinking this would help drive down the price. Does anyone disagree with that? Okay.

I just hope to have a commitment from our folks, from this Committee that we have continued to work on this and that somehow we could add this delinking amendment and get it as part of the package to move forward to actually impact the challenges that we have here already. I guess I got a minute and a half left.

Let's talk about education and nutrition. I will defend Coke and Pepsi for a second. They are going a lot to other more healthy drinks. I see them out there. And more and more, I see young people probably better so than people my age group making healthier choices. Does anybody have any comments on how we can promote that education in a better way?

Dr. TAILLIE. Sure. I mean, I think education is really important and we could do better in our schools by requiring nutrition education, which I believe is not currently required. But we also know that education isn't enough because there are all of these other forces around marketing and pricing, and really the confusing food labeling that makes it complicated.

When you are looking at that product, that sugary drink, and it tells you that it has got 100 percent vitamin C, it can still be hard to understand just how much sugar it has. So, there are other things that we could be doing besides education that would help people make healthier choices. Because we know people want to do that. It is just currently hard to do that even when they have education.

Senator MARSHALL. Okay, thank you so much. I yield back.

The CHAIR. Let me just briefly respond to Senator Marshall. I think you are aware that I consider the high cost of prescription drugs to be one of the great crises facing our healthcare system.

We are going to have to take on 1,800 well-paid lobbyists from the pharmaceutical industry here and all of the campaign contributions that they make. This ain't easy. But I think for the sake of diabetes and so many other illnesses, it should be a major priority of this Committee, and I look forward to working with you to make that happen.

Senator Hassan, I believe, is next.

Senator HASSAN. Thank you, Mr. Chair and Ranking Member Cassidy for this hearing. Thank you to our witnesses for being here today. Really helpful testimony. I want to start with a question to you, Dr. Lipska.

Last year, three major insulin companies announced that they would limit the cost of insulin to $35 a month for all patients. However, we have heard that patients may not actually be getting that discount at the pharmacy counter. In August, Senator Smith and I wrote a letter to Eli Lilly, Novo Nordisk, and Sanofi asking how their companies will ensure that patients can get insulin at this lower price.

The responses from the companies confirm that many patients have to navigate a complex system of manufacturer coupons and online applications in order to access low cost insulin. While these programs allow drug makers to say that their insulin is low cost, it can be really nearly impossible for patients to navigate.

What are you hearing from your patients about the affordability of insulin and other diabetes medications?

Dr. LIPSKA. Thank you for this question. It is so important, and this is why I am here. I heard that the companies announced their cuts. I heard them give you their word, right, and my patients are not getting $35 insulin.

I thought initially, maybe they are doing something wrong. Let me try it. Let me try to print out the coupon. I asked my nurses in the Yale Diabetes Center, are you paying $35? Are you commercially insured? Are you getting this deal?

No, they are not either. So, I don't know. The system is really— it is really difficult to navigate, that is true. But we are savvy at the Yale Diabetes Center, and we can't get that deal.

Senator HASSAN. Well, that is very helpful and something that we all need to follow-up on, obviously. And I appreciate your work in this area. Dr. Kowalski, I wanted to turn to you and thank you and the JDRF for the important work you are doing to advance breakthrough treatments, and 1 day, a cure for type 1 diabetes.

In particular, you mentioned some of these clinical trials on one type of cell therapy, and Dr. Cassidy did too, called islet therapy, has been really promising. This therapy, along with bio-fabrication, is being researched and developed in New Hampshire.

I would invite the Chair and Ranking Member to New Hampshire to see our bio-fabrication center and could remove the need for insulin injections for some patients. Dr. Kowalski, I would like you to speak to the impact that this breakthrough therapy could have on patients with diabetes.

I would also like the Chair and Ranking Member to consider follow-up hearings or work on making sure that the FDA has the approval pathways they need for some of this groundbreaking research.

Dr. KOWALSKI. Excellent. Thank you for the question, Senator Hassan. And I was fortunate to be in Portsmouth at a groundbreaking for a cell manufacturing facility that Vertex is building. Cell therapies have the potential for me to take off my pump, and it gives me incredible excitement.

For years I mentioned cell therapies have provided a pathway to the cures, but they have required somebody to donate a pancreas upon death. We now have the ability to make insulin producing cells from stem cells.

The 8 million people in the United States on insulin could benefit from these tremendous advancements. And Senator Marshall said the Committee hasn't made an impact. They have, you have. The advancements funded by STP to have brought us to the cusp. We are in human trials right now. People are coming off insulin.

The first patient has been off insulin for 2 years now. It is absolutely amazing. So, the continued support here is to drive this toward what we are calling it, an immunosuppression free version, and that is where further research is needed.

But the potential is massive. I truly believe I will be cured in my lifetime, as well my brother, who lives with type 1 diabetes, and this funding is critical to get us there.

Senator HASSAN. Thank you. One more question for you, Dr. Lipska, before my time is up. As we have heard today, new evidence shows that some diabetes drugs such as Ozempic appear to improve other conditions, such as obesity and heart disease.

However, with higher demand for these medications, I am hearing from constituents with diabetes who are experiencing really long delays to get their prescriptions filled. So, how can Congress ensure that all populations that can benefit from this medication have access to it?

Dr. LIPSKA. That is a very important question. Yes, I am seeing patients, my patients who come in previously well-controlled, uncontrolled diabetes because they are not able to access their medication. So, the supply issue is important, but there is also really important shortages because of the price.

Senator HASSAN. Right.

Dr. LIPSKA. And I think that is where this Committee can really help to ensure that patients can afford these drugs, which are transformative, but not if you cannot take it.

Senator HASSAN. Thank you very much. I yield, Mr. Chair.

The CHAIR. Senator Cassidy.

Senator CASSIDY. I will defer to Senator Budd.

Senator BUDD. Thank the Ranking Member. Thank the Chair, and the witnesses for being here today, including, I think, one from North Carolina.

Glad to have you all here. So, back in November, so not too long ago, The Wall Street Journal reported on a phenomenon where pharmacy benefit managers, PBMs, they favor drugs with higher list prices.

I think Senator Marshall mentioned this phenomenon. For example, one particular brand of insulin sells at $274 per vial, while an unbranded counterpart sells at only $25 per vial. Now, according to the Wall Street Journal, half as many Americans have insurance coverage for the less expensive product, as for the higher priced brand, which accounts for about 61 percent of the prescriptions.

Now, this is important because the PBMs that are in there, they preferred coverage for the higher priced medications because they are reimbursed on percentage of the list price. So, the proposal that Senator Marshall discussed on delinking PBM reimbursement from the list price, I think that would go a long way in realigning incentives to best serve the interest of the patients.

Now, a paper published by the American Enterprise Institute makes clear that the list price, and I believe the Chair mentioned list prices when he was referring to some anti-obesity drugs that were $12,000 or so, but I don't think the list price is really the best way to look at that, and that is not the best indicator of their true cost.

Specifically, the study reveals that the rebates that manufacturers pay to those PBMs on anti-obesity medication can be as high as 80 percent of the list price. So, I ask unanimous consent to submit the paper for record.

The CHAIR. Without objection.

[The following information can be found on page 59 in Additional Material:]

Senator BUDD. Thank you, Chairman. Thank you. So, the question. Dr. Kowalski—again, thank you for being here. And again, I appreciate your presence in my State of North Carolina. You are making an impact there and a lot of friends affected by this in similar situation to you.

Natalie, thank you for sharing the story of your daughter, Nadia. So, the insulin of 100 years ago, they are not the same insulin that patients are utilizing today, as I understand. There have been countless innovations with insulin, auto injectors, longer lasting insulin, and some of the references you mentioned.

Dr. Kowalski, could you speak to how public, private partnerships have contributed to some of these advancements?

Dr. KOWALSKI. No, this has been an incredibly important field. When my brother was diagnosed in 1977 and I was diagnosed in 1984, we used to count pig insulin. It was really, really difficult to manage, incredibly unpredictable.

We have seen advancement over advancements in insulin, making insulin easier to use, more effective, and driving better outcomes. Today's insulins are not good enough, and I think this is the balance between innovation and access. JDRF believes we need to continue to innovate in better and better insulins.

For example, we have funded what are called glucose responsive insulins that would only work when your body needs them. These would be transformative. That said, an insulin that is generic and off the patent for many years needs to be accessible.

No one with type 1 diabetes should go without insulin. You die. If you took away my insulin pump, I would die within a week. So, this rationing of insulin is an unacceptable outcome in the United States of America.

This is a balance that we need to strike. But the advancements that continue are critically important. We know the average person with diabetes right now in the United States is not achieving their goals. We need to do better.

Senator BUDD. Appreciate you being here. I yield the floor.

The CHAIR. Thank you, Senator Budd.

Senator Smith.

Senator SMITH. Thank you, Chair. Thanks very much for this hearing, and thanks to all of you for being here. I want to just put a note on what Senator Hassan was asking about related to how people can get access to this, what seems like mythical $35 insulin.

I hear from Minnesotans every single day who tell me that they are rationing this medicine that keeps them alive. And then we have these big companies come in and tell us, oh, it's not us. We are doing everything that we possibly can. We are trying to—we are making our products available. And I don't believe it. I don't think that is what is happening.

Mr. Chair, I think that this is completely unacceptable and obviously it just pisses me off. I really appreciate your testimony about how food is being engineered by these big food companies to be addictive and the impact that has on people's health, their physical health, their mental health. It is pervasive.

I also have been really encouraged by some of the preliminary results that we are seeing for around enrolling diabetic or pre-diabetic patients in food as medicine initiatives. On the other hand, when you actually are consuming real food, it has a big impact on the quality of your health.

These studies, as I understand it, are showing decreases in A1C levels, increases in food security, and improvements in self-management of diabetes. So, Dr. Taillie and Dr. Gearhardt, could you talk a little bit about this? What is the potential of this?

What is the correlation between access to healthy foods and the risk of diabetes, and what should we be doing to take down some of the barriers that make it difficult for providers to support that kind of therapy?

Dr. GEARHARDT. Thank you so much for this really important question. We are actually doing work in my lab right now taking our food as medicine perspective. We have funding from the Eisenberg Family Depression Center at the University of Michigan.

Again, I am seeing as a clinical psychologist just this huge mental health epidemic in adolescents and teens. And we know that the majority of teens, teens are maybe getting more calories from ultra-processed foods than any other developmental stage young children or adults.

Yet we are seeing that when you can move people to real, nourishing whole foods, that it doesn't just help improve their physical health, but their mental well-being. And so, we are actually doing a trial to work with a company Fresh and Lean, to deliver affordable, convenient, minimally processed, ready to go meal packages for people as a potential treatment for depression.

I think we need to think not just about cost and protecting against marketing, but part of what ultra-processed foods do is they are super convenient. They have been designed so you can just pour in your mouth while you are driving your car—and cheap. And so, thinking about ways to make nutritious nourishing food convenient, accessible, and affordable so it can compete with these hyper palatable foods is key.

Senator SMITH. Thank you.

Dr. TAILLIE. The food is medicine data so far are very promising. It shows that it reduces food insecurity, increases intake of fruits and vegetables, and reduces A1C, so that is great. From a prevention perspective though, it means that somebody still has to get sick and access the health care system in order to get those pre scriptions. And in an ideal world, we would see that people had access to those foods as part of their daily lives before they develop obesity or diabetes.

Senator SMITH. I really appreciate that. And it gets to a whole other realm of questions that we could be asking if we were on the Ag Committee around challenges with concentration in the food sector, what that means for how people can get food, food deserts in rural communities and urban communities, particularly black and brown communities. There is a lot of work to be done there.

I want to just follow-up on this for a minute more. We know that American Indian and Alaska Native adults are much more likely than white adults to be diagnosed with diabetes. And we also know that the Special Diabetes Program for Native People, which funds community based initiatives, provides access to people to traditional food, native food is really effective because it incorporates traditional practices and traditional foods in combination with clinical interventions.

It seems like there is a correlation between what we are talking about here. Maybe, I just have a few seconds more, Dr. Lipska. Would you like to talk a bit about why this kind of program can be so effective?

Dr. LIPSKA. Absolutely. I actually spent some time working on the Navajo reservation, so I am very familiar with the setting and the rates of diabetes. You know, we have to tailor the foods, so they are culturally appropriate for our patients, and we have to—but I just want to say, I think we have to go really way upstream—I know we are out of time—with these interventions because it is much harder to intervene, as you said, once people already have prediabetes or obesity.

Senator SMITH. Thank you very much. Thanks, Mr. Chair.

The CHAIR. Thank you.

Senator Cassidy.

Senator CASSIDY. Senator Braun, would you like to go?

Senator BRAUN. Thank you. I am ready. This has been a subject of interest for me way before I got to the U.S. Senate. When you are talking about diabetes, drugs, prevention, and remediation, I wrestled with it to where I was at the point of frustration.

There was nothing that you couldn't generally solve in running a business other than health care, which generally ended up how lucky you were that it was only going up 5 to 10 percent each year.

When we were at the point where I could really do something about it large enough to self-insure, did three simple things. No. 1, I realized none of my employees were health care consumers.

They were the inelastic demands of remediation, generally wanting the plan to pay for everything. And in the same way, if your private plan doesn't pay for it, people look to Government to do it. It has created a system that has given us a bizarre kind of cross purpose where it doesn't jibe with what works in most other markets. What I did, they became health care consumers.

I gave them every wellness tool, including a free biometric screening. I didn't coddle them. You were going to pay more if you wouldn't take that. And you know what it has done? It has lowered health care costs. Not—we have been doing that 15 years and have not had a premium increase.

I would like Dr. Lipska and maybe Dr. Kowalski, how much of what we are talking about here is part of a broken system that is now driven mostly by huge hospitals that love opaqueness, no transparency, and insurance companies that have gone way beyond indemnification to where they are in on everything, and they grab roughly 15 percent of the health care dollar that is purely administrative.

We are talking about things, I think, on the side of how you fix diabetes and other chronic ailments. What about fixing the system itself? I would love for you, Dr. Lipska, to weigh in, and then Dr. Kowalski.

Dr. LIPSKA. Thank you for that question. I agree with you that our system is broken.

In terms of how do we fix this for diabetes in particular, to prevent diabetes, to prevent obesity, I think we—the health care system needs to serve the needs of the patients who develop these conditions, but I think we have to, again, go upstream from the health care system in order to prevent people from getting sick in the first place.

I think that is critical. That is going to save us money and in the long run to keep people healthy. And I think that is upstream from the health care system.

Dr. KOWALSKI. So, I will just make a quick statement because I am going to come in with a research perspective. But start by saying we are talking a lot about obesity and diet, that being obese does not mean you are going to get diabetes.

Sometimes I worry we stigmatize people with type 2 diabetes by saying, and some of our colleagues said this, but you just stop eating and you will get diabetes. This is a genetically inherited disease, so——

Senator BRAUN. And I know that. I am asking about the framework within which you would like to see that we address it and many other things.

Dr. KOWALSKI. Absolutely. So, when we think at JDRF, our mission statement is accelerating life changing breakthroughs to cure, prevent better treat T1D and its complications.

I always take those words very literally and significantly, meaning your life has not changed if you don't have access to better care. And if the system provides barriers, as Senator Sanders said, to drugs that could improve your care and your life and your health, then we haven't succeeded in our mission.

Senator BRAUN. And I agree with that. And I think that is a particularity that will weigh in to be helpful. Let me tell you what I think is a solution to this and the extremely high cost of health care, access and all of it. And proud to say that later today, Senator Sanders and I will be introducing a bill called the Healthcare Price Transparency Act.

I have been working on this for the 5-years I have been in the Senate, and I think it is the umbrella that finally takes us to solutions for this and many other things. Briefly, let me tell you what some of the things it is going to do. It is going to require machine readable files of all negotiated rates and cash prices between plans and providers, not estimates.

It is going to require pricing data standards, including all billing codes for services. It is going to require actual prices for 300 shoppable services, with all services by 2025. It is going to require a testing by executives that all prices are accurate and complete.

It is going to prevent preemption of state price transparency rules, codify the transparency coverage rule, and it is going to provide group health plans the right to access, audit, and review claims and counter data.

Thank you, Senator Sanders and Senator Smith for being on it. I hope to get all Republicans and Democrats on a bill that will fix many aspects of health care.

The CHAIR. Thank you, Senator Braun. Senator Hickenlooper.

Senator HICKENLOOPER. Thank you, Mr. Chair. I thank all of you for being here. I have got a few questions, so I am going to hope you can be very concise. This morning, we have discussed what more we need to do to address upstream causes of obesity that are leading to higher rates of diabetes in our Country.

It is particularly important that we think about what we can do early on to ensure a fewer of our kids end up with type 2 diabetes. In addition to nutrition, one major tool, which has been talked about somewhat, to improve overall health and wellness is access to green spaces and outdoor activity.

Green spaces and getting kids into outdoor recreation can help promote the kind of lifestyle that keeps kids healthy. One in three Americans, including 28 million children, don't have access to green space within a half a mile. We are working on legislation to create a Federal Office of Outdoor Recreation, which will help ensure equitable access to recreation in all communities.

Let's start with Dr. Gearhardt and Dr. Taillie. Can you discuss the benefit that physical activity with healthy eating, along with healthy eating, can have in delaying or preventing the onset of type 2 diabetes?

Dr. GEARHARDT. So, we see that physical activity and nature can play a big role in our overall mental health and well-being. We do see that the role of nutrition and diet can kind of swamp some of those effects.

But I think you are right that it has really got to be multi-pronged and multifaceted, and we need to take holistic views, but also invest our energy and resources where it is going to make the biggest bang for our buck.

Dr. TAILLIE. Yes, to build on that. The diabetes prevention program showed that the combination of physical activity and diet changes were tremendously effective at preventing type 2 diabetes.

But at the same time, going back to Senator Sanders showing us that can of Coke, we know that it is really, really easy to drink a can of Coke, and that would require exercising, running a mile and a half to offset that can of Coke.

It is really important to, in my view, really prioritize nutrition coupled, of course, with physical activity to promote overall fitness. Senator HICKENLOOPER. Great. Thank you so much. Community

health centers place an emphasis on integrated care models, take a comprehensive approach to patient care, focusing not only on treatment but prevention, nutrition, exercise, other social determinants of health.

We have seen some compelling data on this Committee that shows community health centers are more successful at helping patients with hypertension and diabetes control these issues, which really is remarkable because community health centers are more and more dealing with complex chronic conditions.

Dr. Lipska, what can other health care providers learn from community health centers and their approach to caring for a diabetes patients?

Dr. LIPSKA. Thank you. And I think it has to do a lot with the fact that community health centers take that holistic population view as opposed to the rest of health care, which often takes care of the patient in front of you, bill for the service, and then that is it, right.

I think that if we have these systems where you are responsible for the care of the population of patients, you are going to put more emphasis on prevention of disease rather than just treatment of complications when they occur. So, I think we can all learn a lot from that. I think that they are doing a great job.

Senator HICKENLOOPER. I agree. Just one other point on that, or separate from that, is consuming these ultra-processed foods like sugary drinks and all these things you have been—we have been talking about are also connected with higher rates of dementia in later in life. I didn't know whether you or any of the others would like to comment on that.

Dr. GEARHARDT. Yes, there has been some people have even started to think a little bit of Alzheimer's and dementia as type 3 diabetes. It has been discussed a bit.

I could say we have done research with the National Poll and Healthy Aging at the University of Michigan that found in older adults, 13 percent endorsed clinically significant signs of addiction in their intake of ultra-processed foods, and that was associated with higher mental health, physical difficulties, and overall tendency to have a lower quality of life.

I think older adults are a really key population whose increase of ultra-processed foods has been increasing remarkably over the last couple of decades.

Senator HICKENLOOPER. Got it. Great. Thank you. And just very quickly, Ms. Stanback, the National Institute of Diabetes and Digestive and kidney diseases at NIH funds this critical research across the country.

University of Colorado, a Denver diabetes research center with this important support, is spearheading research into type 1 and type 2 diabetes. They also run a program to recruit young faculty into diabetes related research.

Your experience, first with your brother and then with your daughter Nadia, highlights the importance of prioritizing research and making sure future scientists are focusing on treatment. How have the recent medical breakthroughs, even over the course of Nadya's life, changed her experience of living with type 1?

Mrs. STANBACK. Peace of mind. A lot of us are talking about the pharmacy, pharmaceuticals and the medicines that help people with type 1 diabetes, but it also presents a very mental—a serious mental burden that presents in the form of burnout and other things that are detrimental to the health of people living with type 1 diabetes.

Her insulin pump and the CGM gives not only her but me also peace of mind and being able to manage the cumbersome disease. Senator HICKENLOOPER. All right. Thank you. Thank you all. Appreciate you spending time to be here. I yield back to the Chair.

The CHAIR. Thank you. Senator Cassidy.

Senator CASSIDY. We have 5 minutes, so if I interrupt you, I am not being rude—or maybe I am being rude, but that is the reason.

[Laughter.]

Senator CASSIDY. Dr. Kowalski, you mentioned risk factors for type 1 diabetes, but what is there besides genetics? What are the risk factors? Are there other risk factors that we don't know about?

Dr. KOWALSKI. Well, I think you are—so you are hearing that in both forms of diabetes, there is——

Senator CASSIDY. Just type 1.

Dr. KOWALSKI. Okay, but it is genetics and an environmental factor. And if we could find that environmental factor, we could stop this disease.

Senator CASSIDY. So, when you mentioned that we need to focus upon the research, it is just that this has to be developed. It is not that we know it now. You said that we need to study those who have the risk factors, but the principal risk factor would be like Ms. Stanback's family. My gosh, maybe yours because you mentioned your brother having it.

Dr. KOWALSKI. Yes. No, no, there is definitely a genetic component to type 1 diabetes. We know that well. But if you have an identical twin, it is not 100 percent that the second twin, if the first one develops it, will get it.

We have, for example, the STP funding a very, very important study called Teddy that tracks from in utero to adulthood children at high risk. And we are looking at environmental factors that could be triggering the disease. That will stop——

Senator CASSIDY. Let me interrupt you. I graduated from med school in 1983, and they have been talking about it since '83. So, obviously it is pretty difficult to tease out what those environmental factors are.

Dr. KOWALSKI. Very difficult, but we do have a number of candidates that are moving into human clinical trials, and we believe that we will get there.

Senator CASSIDY. That is fantastic. Ms. Stanback, Dr. Lipska mentioned that in her clinic, the workers there have a hard time getting $35 insulin. We know, we are told up here, but we often don't know what we know.

You are the person who has been kind of living with this. So, what is your experience in terms of—and I ask this not knowing the answer, what is your experience in terms of getting affordable insulin?

Mrs. STANBACK. Our insulin is only affordable because we are paying top tier for our private insurance. But I have also not seen it——

Senator CASSIDY. Let me ask you, do you have any insight into what your pharmacy benefit manager—because we have been told pharmacy benefit managers deliberately do not take the low-cost insulin but rather get the higher cost insulin because frankly, the PBMs allegedly make more money by costing you more money. Do you have any insight into that?

Mrs. STANBACK. I don't I just know that we selected the highest tier of the insurance provided by my employer to make sure that we cannot have any ambitions when it comes to choice or selection of insulin.

Senator CASSIDY. That is great. And Dr. Lipska, do y'all have any insight into what Yale does for its PBMs? Because again, this does come up continuously and this is the big rub. Eli Lilly says, hey, listen, we are given it for $35. Yes, there is a tax, there is a dispensing fee, but our cost is $35.

The PBMs allegedly are saying, no, we are going to give you the top dollar and we are not going to take this one. Do you have any— when you inquire about this, do you know whether that extra cost being paid is due to the PBM or to the drug company?

Dr. LIPSKA. That is a great question. I don't know. I honestly haven't been able to get to the bottom of why this happens because it is so difficult.

Senator CASSIDY. So, let me ask then, and this may come to you, it is my understanding that on some of these processed foods, it is fructose more than glucose or sucrose, which is the problem.

That fructose is more quickly absorbed and causes a greater sugar high and kind of the greater sugar low, so therefore you want another hit. Now, again, I haven't looked at this for some time, but is that still kind of the thought?

Dr. LIPSKA. Yes, I think—I don't know if the other panelists want to answer that as well since, again, I treat diabetes, but I am familiar with some of that research and I understand that is true, that fructose does activate those rewards systems.

Senator CASSIDY. Could one of you all answer that quickly, please?

Dr. TAILLIE. That is true. But the high fructose corn syrup that we are consuming is actually very similar to sugar, from a chemical composition perspective.

Senator CASSIDY. The fructose?

Dr. TAILLIE. The main—yes.

Senator CASSIDY. Yes, but the fructose is more quickly absorbed.

Dr. TAILLIE. The main issue is also that we are consuming it via liquid forms, which means that it is much more rapidly digested. And that is true for ultra-processed foods as well. The way that those foods are made means that they are metabolized much more rapidly.

Senator CASSIDY. I get that, yes—the more fiber, the apple juice is absorbed more rapidly than applesauce, which is more rapidly than an apple.

Dr. TAILLIE. Exactly.

Senator CASSIDY. More fiber is slower absorption. But fructose is the independent factor, and it does seem like fructose is a particular issue here, I will just point that out. Ms. Stanback, coming back to you.

Again, we have had these kinds of conversations as regards PBMs. When you change insurance companies, because periodically employers do, are they making you go through a prior authorization process for whatever your daughter's currently on?

The brand new one, no, this didn't work before, but you got to go through it once more just to satisfy our requirements?

Mrs. STANBACK. No, not with our private insurance. It is through my employer.

Senator CASSIDY. Do you have a big employer or a small employer?

Mrs. STANBACK. It is fairly large.

Senator CASSIDY. Do you mind telling us?

Mrs. STANBACK. I work for AMN Healthcare, medical staffing. Senator CASSIDY. Yes. That is a pretty big company. Okay, well,

I am almost out of time, but I thank you all.

The CHAIR. Thank you. Senator Kaine.

Senator KAINE. Thank you, Chair Sanders. And great hearing, great witnesses. I would like to put an unusual document into the record. It is a JDRF 2023 children's Congress scrapbook.

A bunch of students in Virginia who have diabetes told their stories and they are Emory Ellis, Maddie Hawkins, Riley Kitts, Karson Owen, Jack Samples, Jane Vanden Eykel. I think these are worthy testimony.

I just want to read one that was interesting from Maddie Hawkins. She is in a family where mom, dad and her brother, the mother doesn't have diabetes, all the others have type 1 diabetes.

Listen to this. My dad was diagnosed with diabetes before I was even born and my brother diagnosed in 2020, so it is always crazy at my house. There is always some alarm going off, always someone who needs to treat their blood sugar. My mom's goal in life is for all of us to have the same blood sugar at the same time, but that hasn't happened yet. Still, at the end of the day, sharing diabetes creates a sense of camaraderie.

Then there is a picture of the dad and the two kids who share this camaraderie because they have diabetes. I would just like to put that into the record.

The CHAIR. Without objection.

[The following information can be found on page 60 in Additional Material:]

Senator KAINE. And focusing on young people, during the height of the pandemic, Congress provided schools with a lot of flexibilities around meals.

One in five kids in the U.S. live without constant access to adequate food, and this temporary expansion during COVID allowed students, especially those in high need areas, to have much more access to meals that were nutritious.

Now, the pandemic era policies in several states have enacted legislation allowing for universal free school meals. In Virginia, there are currently about 511 schools that have adopted the community eligibility provision where eligible schools can offer meals at no cost to all students.

I am heartened to see this uptick in the CEP in my home state. Dr. Taillie, what impact does the nutritional value of school lunches have on students' health, and what can Congress do to improve health outcomes for kids?

Dr. TAILLIE. School foods are probably the No. 1 way that we could promote healthier diets among kids and ultimately prevent diabetes. Kids consume a third of their daily calories in school, so this is incredibly important.

Universal school meals are critical because it ensures that all kids have access to food. We know that adequate nutrition is not only important for health and growth, but it promotes learning outcomes.

It also means that kids are stigmatized for receiving when only some kids get this benefit. So, in addition to universal school meals, as I said in my testimony, really making sure that our schools are free from corporate food marketing, ultra-processed foods, sugary drinks.

The marketing and advertisement and sales of those products to our kids is currently a major problem, and so reducing or eliminating that would make huge progress.

Senator KAINE. Let me ask another question. I have heard an interesting policy debate, and the question is should SNAP benefits be usable to purchase unhealthy and ultra-processed foods? Those who say yes say you shouldn't have a separate standard for people using a SNAP benefit—pardon, person using dollars and cents.

Those who say that SNAP benefits shouldn't be used, say why would we want to pay tax dollars to enable people to purchase foods that make them sick or kill them? And if SNAP benefits weren't usable for unhealthy foods, the food retailers and grocery stores that are in neighborhoods where there is a high percentage of SNAP recipients would have more of a motive to offer more healthy food options. What do you all think about that debate?

Dr. TAILLIE. Yes, I can weigh in on this. I have tried to do research in the past on this and wasn't able to receive funding. I think it is really important to make sure that people who are using SNAP have dignity and choice.

At the same time, when we think about restricting, I think the clear place where we would start with that is around sugary drinks. I think there is an argument to be made that those may not even be considered as foods.

They provide no nutritional value. And the health harms are so very clear that SNAP is currently not allowed to use for like hot meals or alcohol or things like that, and I could see putting sugary drinks into that category.

Senator KAINE. Are thoughts from other panelists?

Dr. GEARHARDT. I think the problem is that those foods are also—the unhealthy foods are also cheaper, right. So, then your SNAP benefit is going to go potentially a longer way—if you can make those foods, the healthy foods, more affordable, that would make it easier.

Dr. TAILLIE. And beyond restricting, the double up box program is a really effective strategy to instead of saying, well, you can't buy this, to incentivize people to buy fruits and vegetables by giving them more money to do that.

Senator KAINE. Thank you. Mr. Chairman, last I will mention, which isn't really a question, is I know we are talking about doing work on the Older Americans Act next year, and I think there is a lot in this space that really we could do as part of a reauthorization of the Older Americans Act that has been touched on in the testimony earlier and look forward to working with you on that.

The CHAIR. I agree. Okay, Senator Casey.

Senator CASEY. Thank you, Mr. Chairman. I want to thank the panel. And sorry I wasn't here earlier. We had an Aging Committee hearing that I was Chairing that overlapped. So, we have your testimony, and I am—I know that Sara and my team has been here for the whole hearing.

I wanted to thank the witnesses for your testimony, bringing both experience and expertise to these issues. And I know the hearing touched on a number of critical issues relating to diabetes and including the high cost of insulin.

I was one of the, many were co-sponsors of Senator Warnock's bill that proposed a cap on co-payments for insulin in the commercial market at $35 bucks a month. That was similar to what we passed and the Inflation Reduction Act for Medicare Part D beneficiaries. So, I just have two questions, Dr. Kowalski, and I will start with you.

Type 1 diabetes is often perceived as a disease of children and young adults, but as health care for people living with diabetes has improved, it is truly a disease that can affect people a much longer time period throughout their lives, as you know. Are there specific challenges or factors we should consider with respect to older adults with type 1 diabetes? That is the first part of the question.

Then second, are there medical issues that need more research or policy changes specific to the needs of older adults that you would recommend?

Dr. KOWALSKI. Well, the great news is people with Type 1 diabetes are living longer. When I was diagnosed, we were told we were to have significant reduction in lifespan. And my brother and I fortunately are doing well, and many people.

That said, we know that older adults are particularly susceptible to severe hypoglycemia, hypoglycemia unawareness, which kind of called for because falls and broken bones.

Unfortunately, broken bones are another issue in older adults with diabetes. So, that is an area. Reducing hypoglycemia is a big, big priority. As we drive better glucose control, we know that complications of diabetes that have been mentioned by a number of panelists, heart and kidney in particularly, are forestalled but don't go away.

The risk of long-term kidney disease, which is a major driver of CMF's cost, is another area where we are making progress. We have mentioned the benefits of these new drugs. GLP, SGLP inhibitors can reduce diabetic kidney disease and cardiovascular disease, a particular problem in older adults for type 1 and type 2 diabetes. So, this is an opportunity to reduce costs and improve care.

Senator CASEY. Thanks very much, Dr. Taillie—did I pronounce it right? Nutrition for children is obviously fundamental, as so many have made reference to. I introduced a bill that focused on what I believe are what should be the five freedoms for children.

One of them is a freedom from hunger, in addition to health care and education, and so much else that we want to provide our kids. At the end of your written testimony, I think it is on page six, you mention the need for more research into nutrition science. What are some of the current gaps in our knowledge about nutrition, especially as it relates to kids?

Dr. TAILLIE. One of the gaps that we have been talking a lot about is the fact that we still don't have a really good understanding for the biological mechanisms of how ultra-processed foods work. They are such complex substances.

Kevin Hall at DNH did a wonderful trial that was the first step in showing this, but there have been no additional studies to replicate that, to look at this issue in kids, and to really go further— to really isolate what those effects are.

I think that would be the first piece of this. And then the second piece is understanding from a population level perspective, we are not thinking about how to treat these kids, we are trying to think about what policies work more broadly to prevent hunger and also promote healthy diets, because those things often kind of go hand- in-hand.

We have a lot of kids who are hungry and also consuming diets that are really high in sugary drinks and ultra-processed foods.

Senator CASEY. Thanks very much. Thanks, Mr. Chairman.

The CHAIR. Senator Cassidy, you want a brief closing remark?

Senator CASSIDY. Yes. Dr. Kowalski, I know you would agree with me totally, but just for the record, you mentioned that obesity does not necessarily lead to type 2 diabetes, but let's not imply that obesity does not have other problems associated with it.

Hip replacements, joint replacements, heart disease, hypertension, gallstones, what was mentioned earlier about Alzheimer's, on and on and on. And so, I am a big proponent for obesity research.

If the metabolic syndrome is almost always triggered by obesity, and I used to tell my medical students it is a hydra headed monster, and diabetes is one of those but there is many others as well.

I think we need to be asking the NIH and CDC to focus more attention upon obesity in of itself. And I know you agree with that, but just for the record.

Dr. KOWALSKI. I agree.

The CHAIR. That was a brief remark. Good. Let me thank all of our witnesses. I thought a very informative hearing, and I thank all of you for being here.

We have touched on a lot of issues the need for more research in type 1 diabetes and the need to address the crisis, and our kids becoming too heavy and the foods that they are eating, what they are drinking, and the need for affordable treatments.

We covered a lot of territory that I hope this Committee will effectively deal with but thank you all very much for being here. And with that, this is the end of our hearing today, and I—for any Senators who wish to ask additional questions, questions for the record will be due in 10 business days, December 29th at 5.00 p.m.

The Committee stands adjourned. Thank you all.

## Additional Material

### Endocrine Society

The Endocrine Society thanks the Senate Health, Education, Labor, and Pensions (HELP) Committee for conducting this hearing on the diabetes epidemic. We appreciate that the Committee is examining this critical issue, which impacts millions of people across the country. The Endocrine Society is the world's largest and oldest Society representing clinicians and scientists working to treat and research endocrine diseases and disorders. Founded in 1916, the Society represents approximately 18,000 physicians and scientists engaged in the management and research of endocrine disorders. Our membership includes over 11,000 clinicians who are on the front lines in treating diabetes and obesity, which are two of the most common chronic illnesses in the United States. Our member researchers are making significant contributions to the advancement of knowledge in diabetes research, prevention, and treatment and we have prioritized these issues in our policy work.

There is a diabetes crisis in America requiring immediate attention by Congress. Diabetes affects over 38 million people in the United States, which represents 11.6 percent of the U.S. population, and this number continues to increase at an alarming rate. The prevalence rate is even more alarming when broken down by race, ethnicity, and age. Approximately 29.2 percent of people over the age of 65 have diabetes; 16 percent of American Indian and Alaska Natives; 12.5 percent of African Americans; and 10.3 percent of Hispanic Americans have diabetes. No part of the country is immune from diabetes and many of the states represented by Members of this Committee are significantly impacted by this disease. Despite the fact that we know how to effectively treat and manage diabetes, prevent type 2 diabetes, and delay the onset of type 1 diabetes the number of people with diabetes continues to rise and people living with diabetes continue to experience barriers to access to care and affordability of the medicines they require. The Endocrine Society urges theSenate HELP Committee to support and advance the following bipartisan legislation to address the diabetes crisis in our Country today: Reauthorization of the Special Diabetes Program, passage of the INSULIN Act, and passage of the Treat & Reduce Obesity Act.

**Special Diabetes Program**

The Special Diabetes Program (SDP) is a Federal program comprised of two components: the Special Diabetes Program for Type 1 Diabetes and the Special Diabetes Program for Indians (SDPI). Congress created these programs in 1997 to advance research for type 1 diabetes at the National Institute of Diabetes and Digestive and Kidney Disorders (NIDDK) and to provide type 2 treatment and education programs for American Indians and Alaska Natives (AI/AN). SDP continues to receive strong bipartisan support because of the program's many successes. It has delivered groundbreaking research on the artificial pancreas, which has led to the development of commercial devices; research that has resulted in the FDA approval of the first drug that can delay the onset of type 1 diabetes; and the first cellular therapy to treat adults with type 1 diabetes who have reoccurring episodes of dangerously low blood glucose levels. SDP is currently operating on a short-term extension which expires on January 19th. Short-term extensions are extremely harmful to the Program and make it difficult for researchers to map out long-term plans for their research. It also puts the important education and treatment programs for AI/AN communities in jeopardy. *We urge Congress to reauthorize SDP through the end of 2025 at $170 million per-program, per-year, which is a 13 percent increase in current funding.* We were glad to see that the HELP Committee approved S. 1855, the Special Diabetes Program Reauthorization Act in a bipartisan fashion and we urge the Senate to reauthorize SDP before the program expires on January 19, 2024.

## Insulin Affordability

As you know, insulin is a life-saving medication for many people living with diabetes. Unfortunately, despite being over 100 years old, insulin is a medication that continues to be unaffordable for many who rely on it. While the Endocrine Society hears from our members about many different clinical and research issues, the rising out-of-pocket cost of insulin is one causing the greatest concern for our patients. *We urge the Senate to pass S. 1269, the INSULIN Act of 2023, which is bipartisan legislation that would improve insulin affordability and access for the more than 7 million people nationwide who rely on this medication to manage their diabetes.* This legislation, introduced by Senators Jeanne Shaheen (D-NH) and Susan Collins (R-ME), the co-Chairs of the Senate Diabetes Caucus, includes several policies to make insulin more affordable. It would expand the $35 insulin co-pay cap, currently available for people on Medicare, to the private insurance market which would ensure that people on private health plans would pay no more than $35 per month for their insulin. The legislation would also ensure that people who rely on insulin are able to share in insulin rebates and discounts which often go to pharmacy benefit managers and private insurers. Finally, the legislation would promote competition by encouraging the approval of more generic and bio-similar insulins.

## Obesity

While the primary focus of this briefing is on diabetes, it is also important for the Committee to recognize obesity, which is related to diabetes and another costly chronic disease impacting millions of Americans. As you know, people living with obesity are at increased risk of developing type 2 diabetes and many other complications. We are alarmed by the increased prevalence of obesity across the country. Over 42 percent of all U.S. adults and over 19 percent of children are estimated to have obesity in the United States. Obesity has a significant impact on economic costs accounting for $170 billion in higher medical costs each year. It has also impacted our Nation's military readiness and national security. Just over 1 in 3 young adults between the ages of 17 and 24 are too heavy to serve in our military. The management of obesity includes a range of options including lifestyle intervention and pharmacotherapy. Unfortunately, there are restrictions currently in place which prevent millions of Americans from accessing obesity treatment and care. Most notably, Medicare is currently prohibited by statute from covering FDA approved anti-obesity medications. Research shows that adding pharmacotherapy for weight management results in increased weight loss and overall improved health. Because Medicare is unable to cover these medications, which are scientifically proven to be effective, many private insurers also do not cover them because Medicare often sets the standard on what is covered. We urge the Senate to pass S. 2407, the Treat and Reduce Obesity Act (TROA), which would allow Medicare to cover FDA approved anti-obesity medications and also make it easier for Medicare beneficiaries to access Intensive Behavioral Therapy (IBT), which is an effective lifestyle intervention for obesity. We encourage you to work with your colleagues on the Finance Committee to advance this important legislation.

We commend the Committee for taking time to discuss this critically important issue of diabetes and the impact it has on millions of Americans. We urge you to work swiftly to pass bipartisan legislation that prioritizes the groundbreaking research that continues to be done and ensures access and affordability for people living with diabetes and obesity. Our patients living with diabetes cannot wait longer. The Endocrine Society would like to work with you by providing information, having our member diabetes experts be a resource to you, and sharing our recommendations as you consider how to address this important public health issue. Please do not hesitate to contact Rob Goldsmith, Director of Advocacy and Policy, at rgoldsmith@ endocrine.org for more details.

## Estimating the Cost of New Treatments for Diabetes and Obesity

The rising popularity of drugs to treat obesity and diabetes, including Ozempic, has focused attention on their costs. However, existing research has incompletely characterized prices by focusing on only discounted list prices. We estimate that net prices received by drugmakers are 48–78 percent lower than list prices. In effect, we document a large difference between net payments to manufacturers and the prices faced by some consumers who pay list prices, even after we adjust for currently available coupons from manufacturers. We conclude by highlighting uncertainty surrounding future prices of drugs in this class and policy implications.

The introduction of glucagon-like pcptide–1 agonists (CLP–1s), which include drugs such as Ozempic, represents a milestone in the treatment of diabetes and obesity. Clinical evidence suggests that diabetes products can help control blood sugar among diabetics, lower weight, reduce cardiovascular events and ease symptoms of heart failure.[23]

With mounting evidence of clinical benefit, these drugs have attracted understandable levels of policy attention, much of it focused on their cost. Recent projections suggest revenue for GLP-1s could reach $100 billion annually over the next decade (Erman 2023).

The majority of news coverage and research on these drugs has focused on their publicly available list price.[24] While list prices arc relevant for some patients, prior research has shown that this is often a highly incomplete summary of typical transaction prices in the U.S. This reflects the relatively opaque use of ‘‘rebates’’ and other discounts, which alter the prices paid for branded drug products.

In this report, we aim to characterize the prices of these drugs more completely. In doing so, we hope to give researchers, policymakers, and journalists a fuller and more accurate understanding of these products' current costs.

---

[23] For a discussion of evidence on glucagon-like peptide-1 agonists (GLP-1s), see Herman (2023). For recent evidence on semaglutide's effect on major adverse cardiovascular events, see Novo Nordisk (2023). For recent evidence on semaglutide's effect on heart failure, see Kosiborod et al. (2023).

[24] For example, see Amin et al. (2023) and Cirruzzo and Leonard (2023).

Children's Congress

JDRF

SENATOR

# TIM KAINE

Meet your JDRF 2023 Children's Congress Delegates

VIRGINIA

Emory Ellis

Maddie Hawkins

Riley Kitts

Karson Owen

Jack Samples

Jane Vanden Eykel

**My name is Emory Ellis, and I am excited to be a delegate from Virginia at the 2023 JDRF Children's Congress! I live in Ashburn, VA and am a rising senior at Stone Bridge High School.**

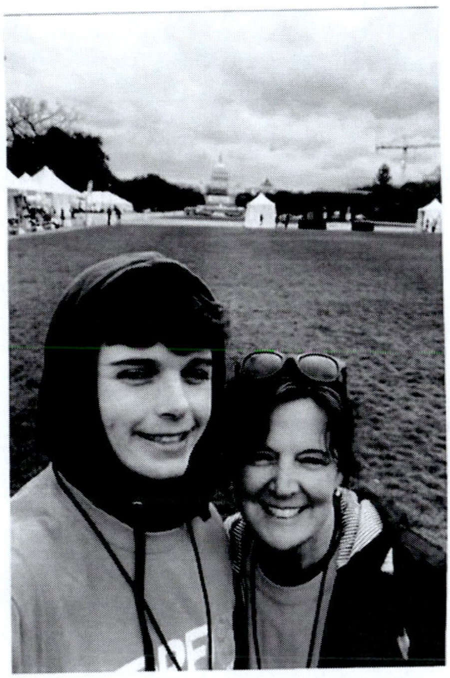

**I was diagnosed with Type 1 Diabetes on March 5, 2018 when I was 12 years old. My diagnosis came a year after my older brother, Declan, was diagnosed and a year before my older sister, Annie, was diagnosed. Since my brother had been living with T1D for a year, we were able to recognize the symptoms early enough to keep me from going into DKA at diagnosis.**

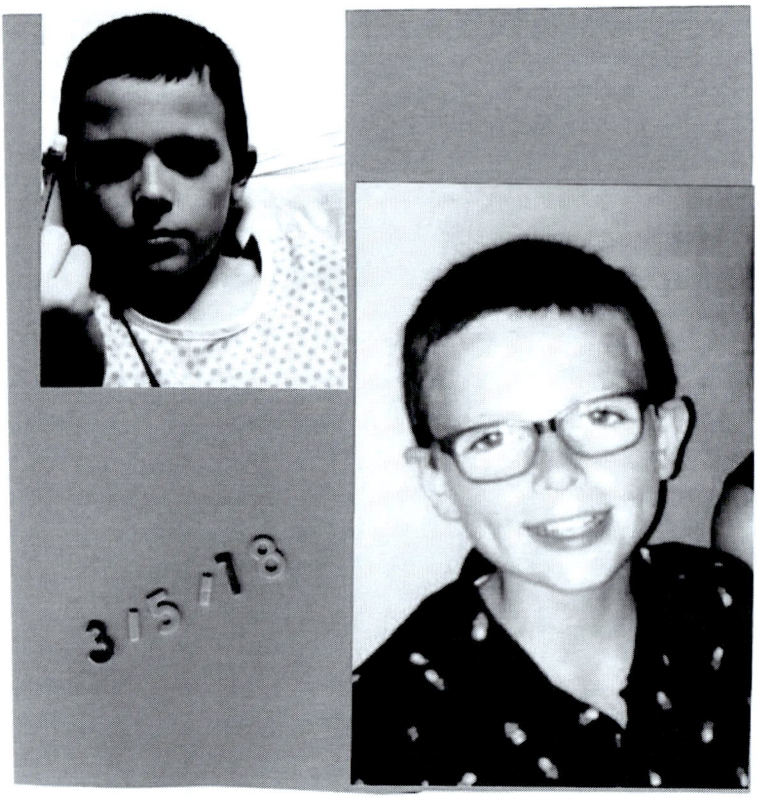

I knew I wanted to use a continuous glucose monitor. I saw how much easier it was for Declan to manage his highs and lows when he got his CGM, and our Dexcoms come with an app that lets my mom know if we have an urgent low or if our blood sugars go too high.

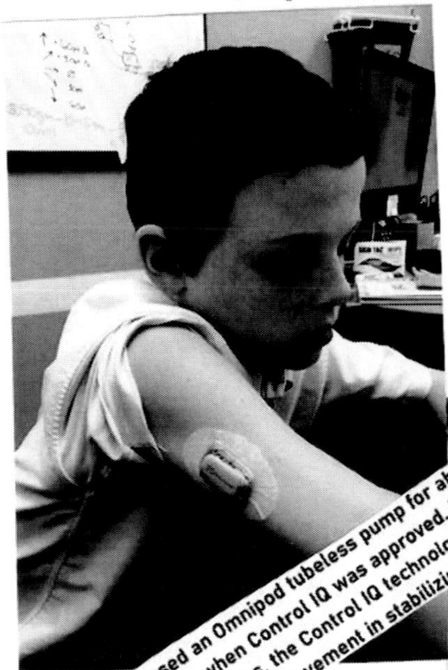

I also used an Omnipod tubeless pump for about 3 years. I switched to a tSlim pump when Control IQ was approved. Even though I liked not having wires and tubes, the Control IQ technology is really helpful and a huge improvement in stabilizing my blood sugar.

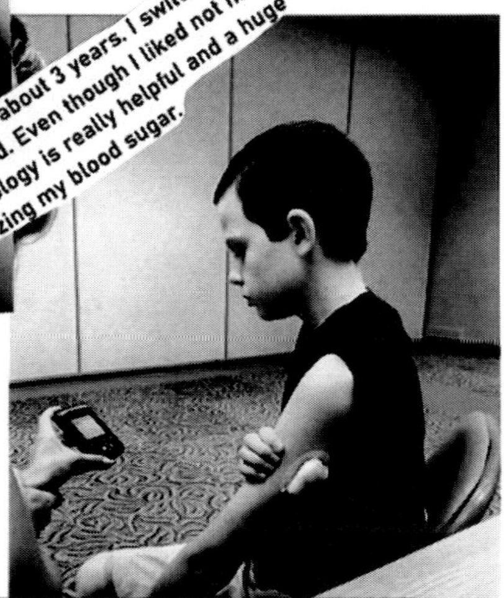

Every new advancement in technology means a healthier, safer life for people with T1D. I hope that one day soon the technologies that keep us safe will be accessible to everyone living with T1D.

I am thankful to have siblings who understand what it is to live with T1D. We support each other and help each other through the challenges that come with living with T1D.

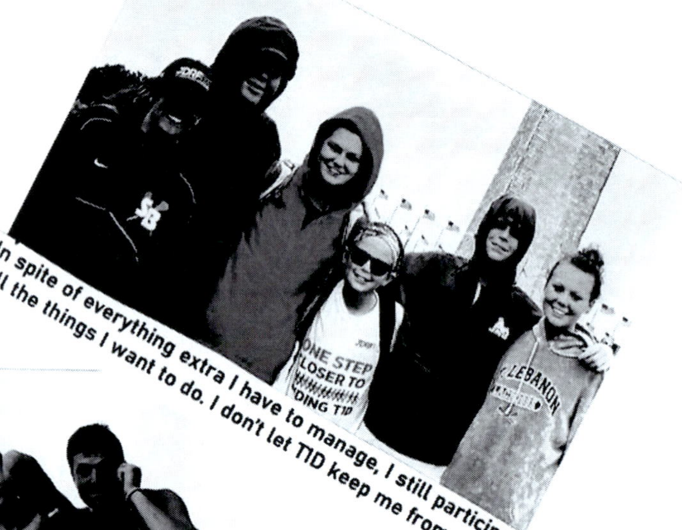


In spite of everything extra I have to manage, I still participate in all the things I want to do. I don't let T1D keep me from anything.

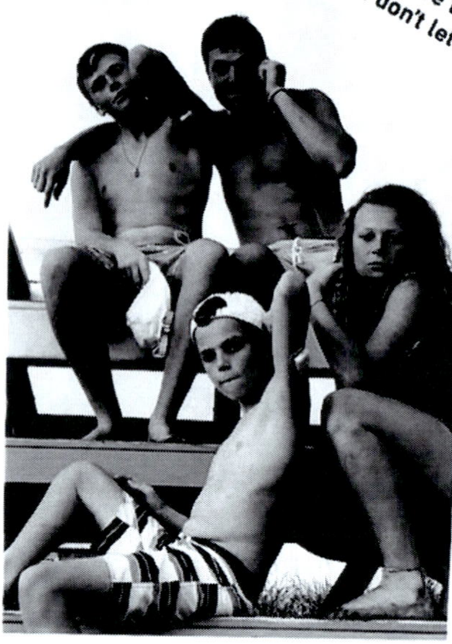

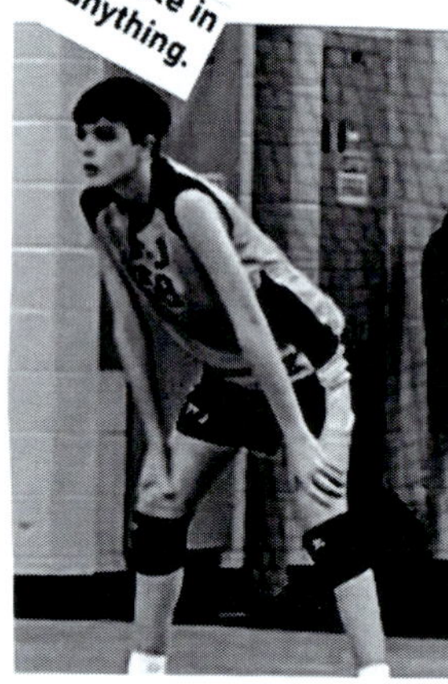

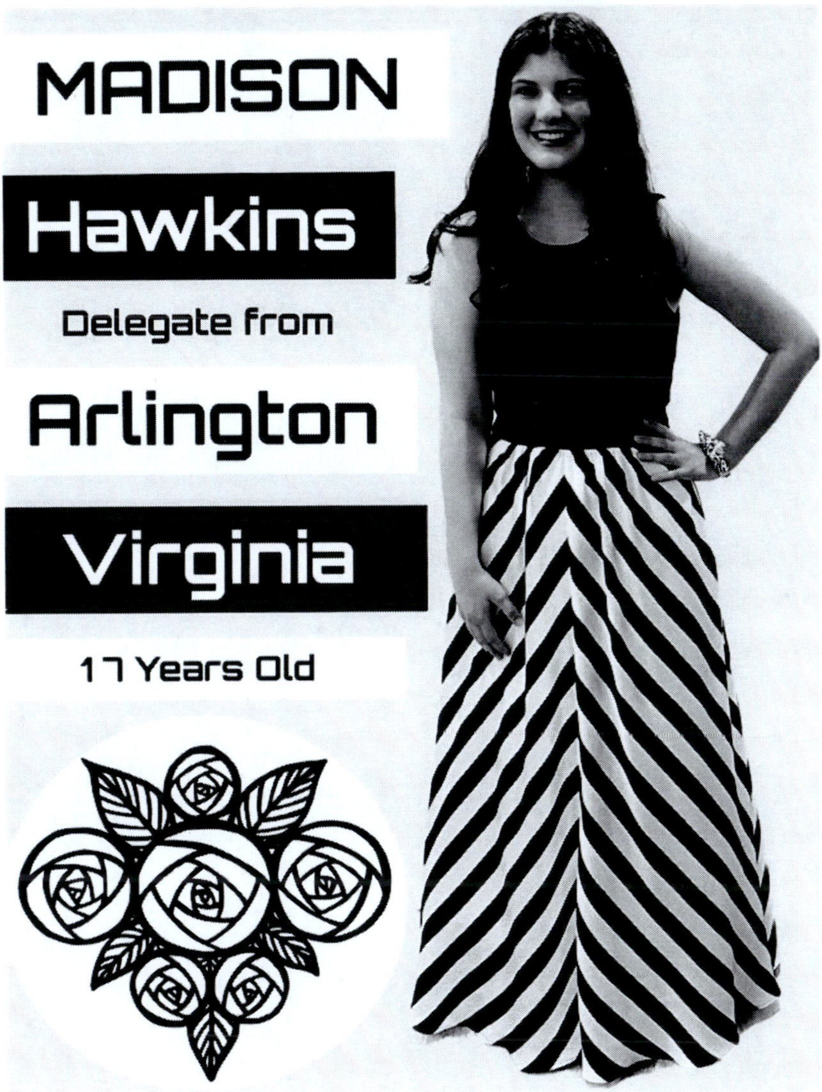
MADISON
Hawkins
Delegate from
Arlington
Virginia
17 Years Old

On February 19th, 2009, a month after my 3rd birthday, I got diagnosed with Type 1 Diabetes. I don't remember much about that day, nor the following months, but I do remember my dad sitting with me in my hospital bed. My dad had diabetes as well, and he told me that everything would be alright, words which have stuck with me forever.

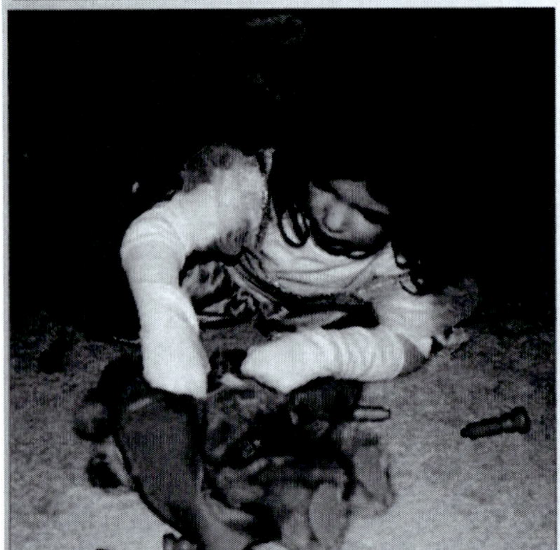

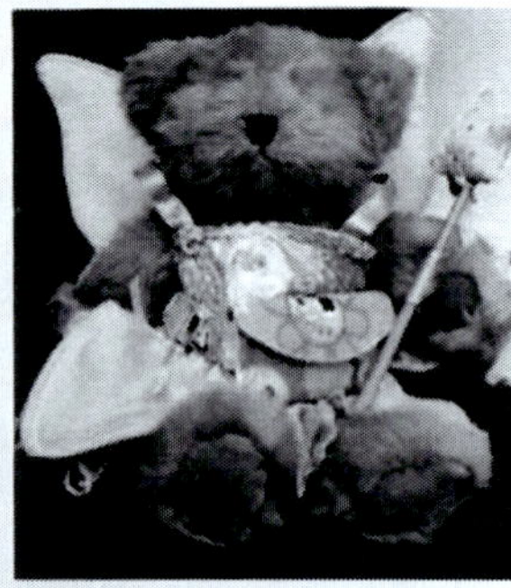

At the hospital, I got a JDRF bear, named Madison Bear. She went through all the same trials as me, from receiving shots (shown in the picture) to getting a new pump.

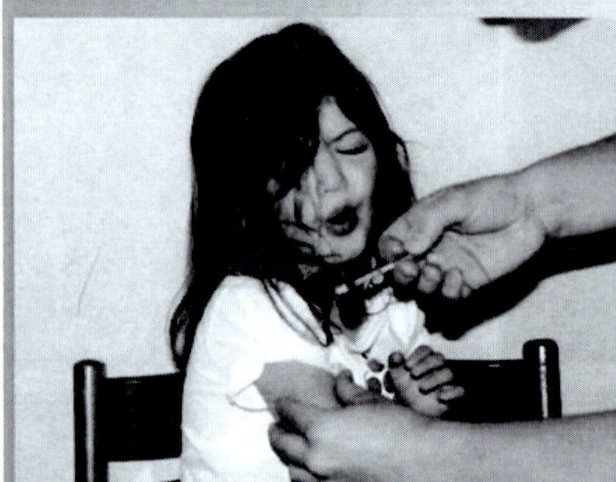

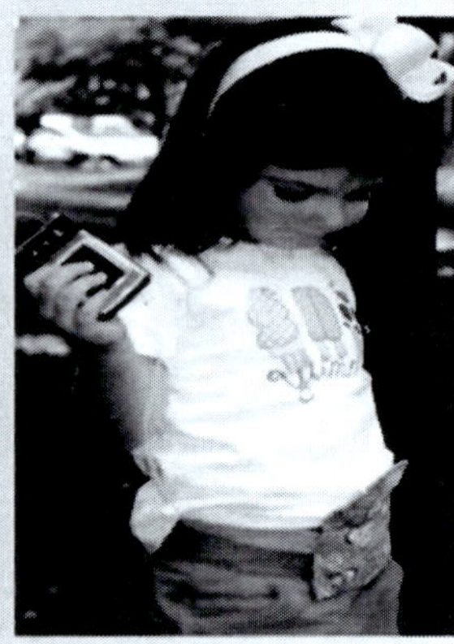

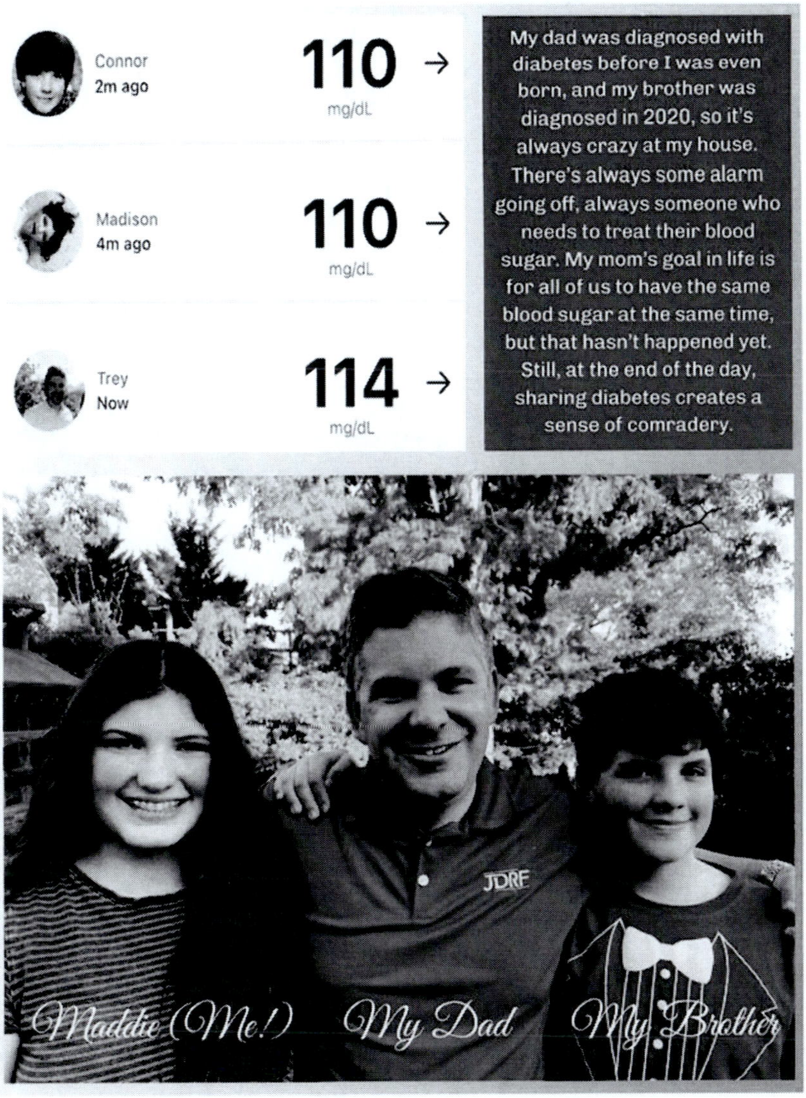
Connor
2m ago
110 →
mg/dL
Madison
4m ago
110 →
mg/dL
Trey
Now
114 →
mg/dL
My dad was diagnosed with diabetes before I was even born, and my brother was diagnosed in 2020, so it's always crazy at my house. There's always some alarm going off, always someone who needs to treat their blood sugar. My mom's goal in life is for all of us to have the same blood sugar at the same time, but that hasn't happened yet. Still, at the end of the day, sharing diabetes creates a sense of comradery.
JDRF
Maddie (Me!)
My Dad
My Brother

I've participated in many clinical trials over the years, from week long summer camps to many months of wearing the same version of a new insulin pump. I know I can make a difference when I participate

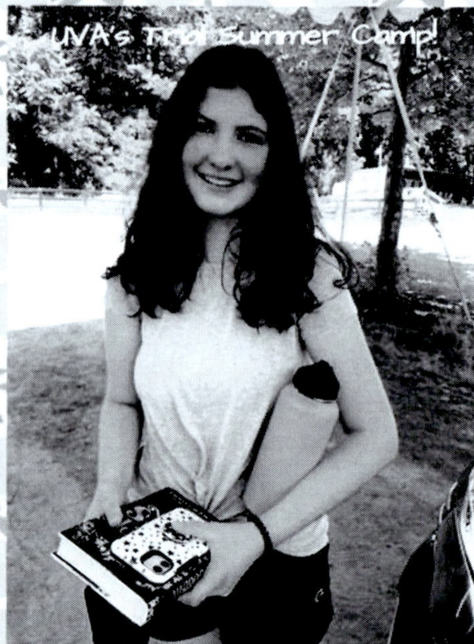


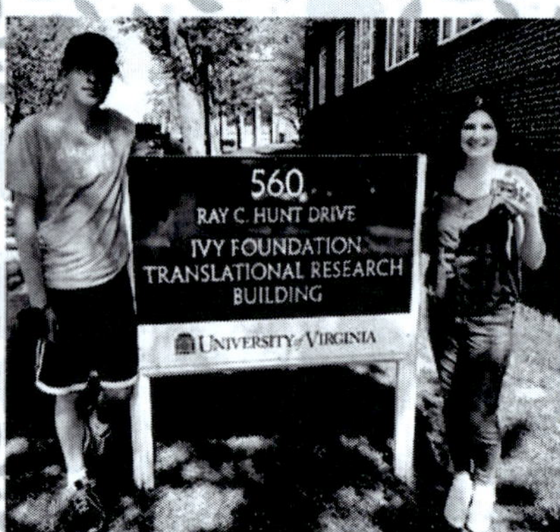


In fact, I'm currently in a trial right now at UVA! This is a picture of me and my brother with a new version of the a Tandem pump. We are testing out new features that will come out in a few years.

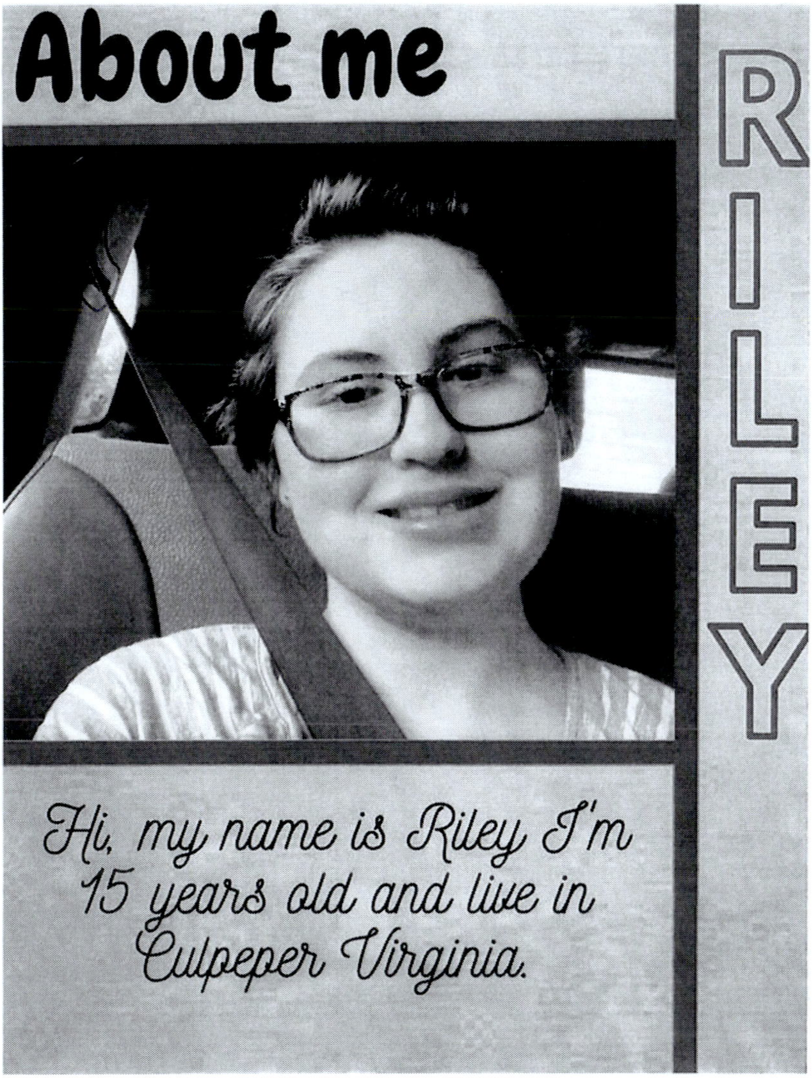
About me
RILEY
Hi, my name is Riley I'm
15 years old and live in
Culpeper Virginia.

# My diagnosis

Before Diagnosis

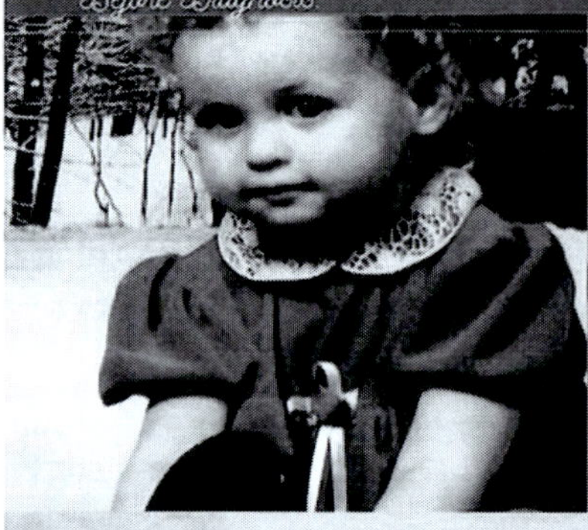

After diagnosis

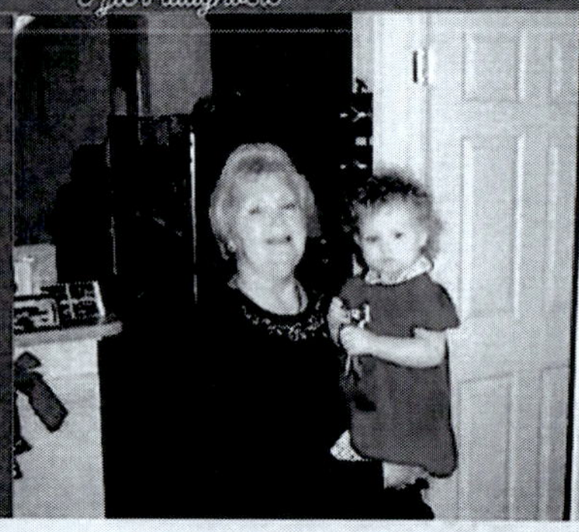

I don't remember my diagnosis, since I was 21 months. Ive been told that I was constantly thirsty and wetting through my diapers. I was also extremely grumpy and was usually a happy toddler. My parents took me to the doctor, and my blood sugar was too high to read on the meter. I then spent several days in ICU.

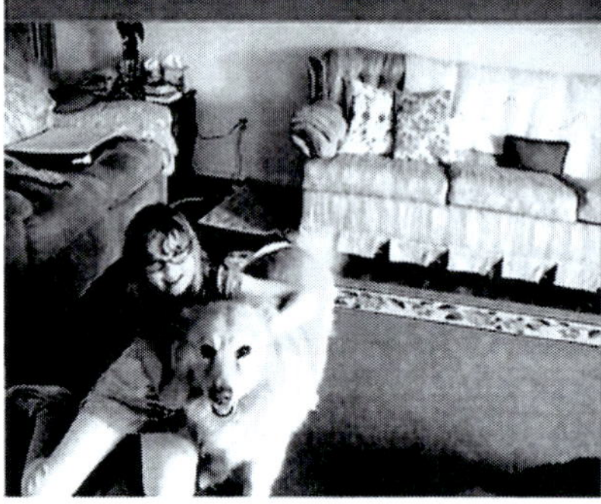

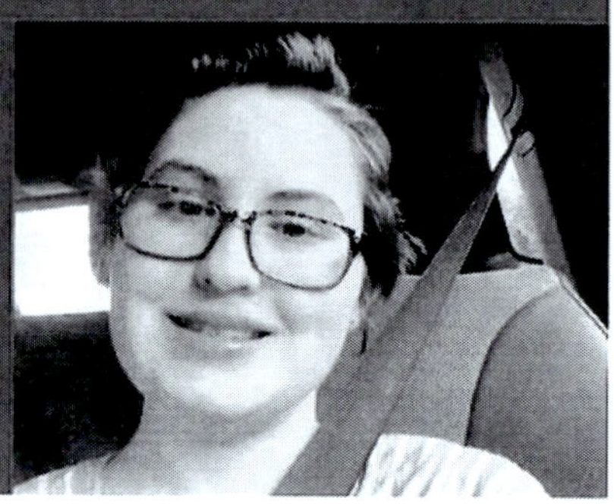

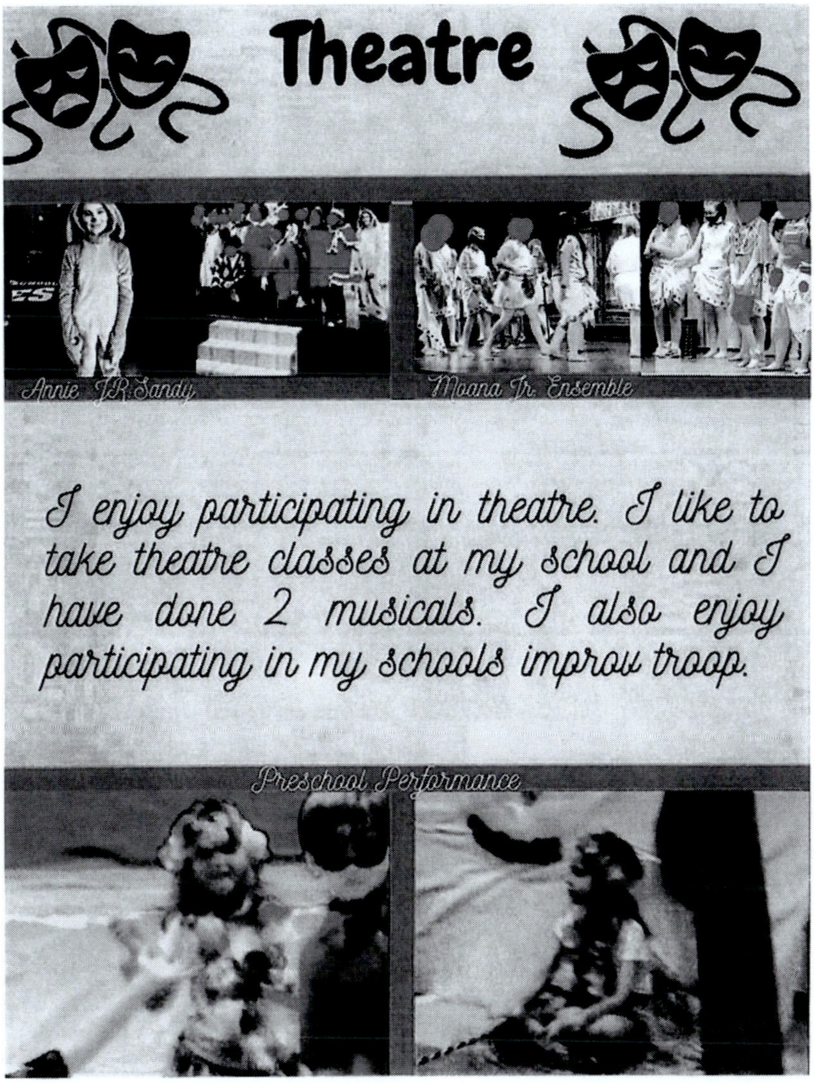
Theatre
Annie JR Sandy
Moana Jr. Ensemble
I enjoy participating in theatre. I like to take theatre classes at my school and I have done 2 musicals. I also enjoy participating in my schools improv troop.
Preschool Performance

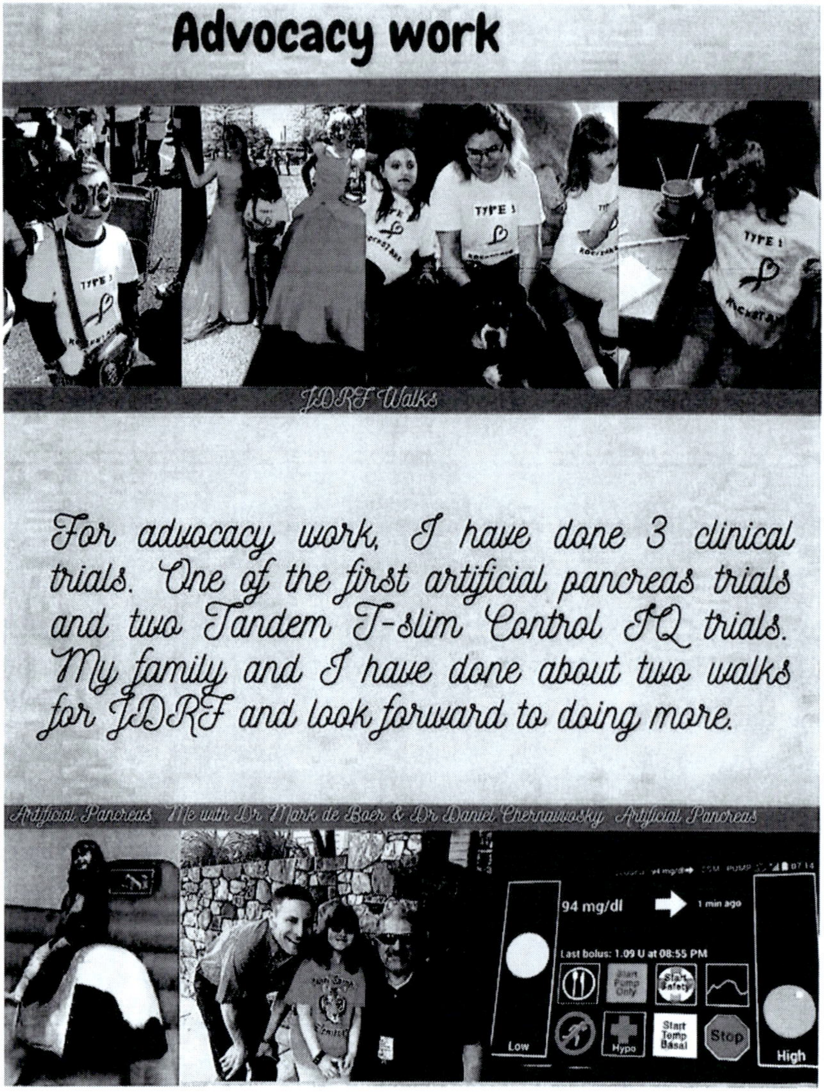
Advocacy work
JDRF Walks
For advocacy work, I have done 3 clinical trials. One of the first artificial pancreas trials and two Tandem T-slim Control IQ trials. My family and I have done about two walks for JDRF and look forward to doing more.
Artificial Pancreas
Me with Dr Mark de Boer & Dr Daniel Chernavvosky
Artificial Pancreas
94 mg/dl
1 min ago
Last bolus: 1.09 U at 08:55 PM
Start Pump Only
Start Safety
Low
Hypo
Start Temp Basal
Stop
High

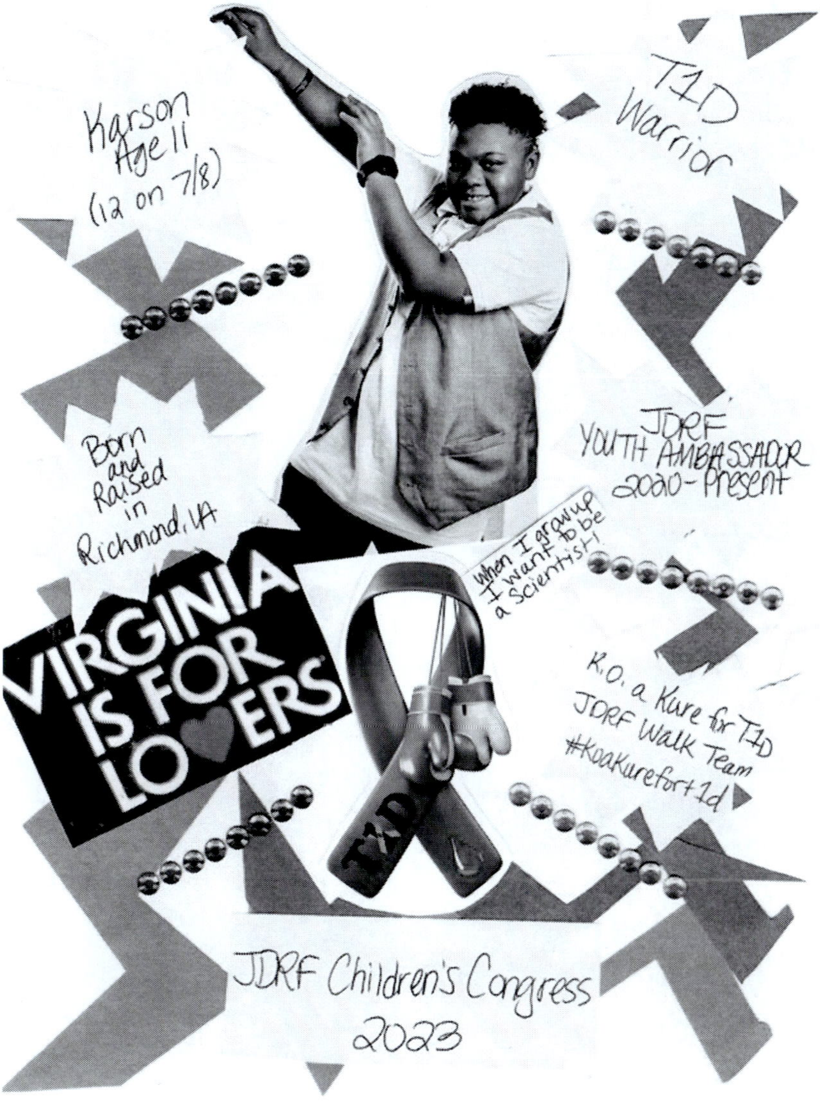
Karson
Age 11
(12 on 7/8)
T1D
Warrior
Born
and
Raised
in
Richmond, VA
JDRF
YOUTH AMBASSADOR
2020-Present
When I grow up
I want to be
a scientist!
VIRGINIA
IS FOR
LOVERS
T1D
K.O. a Kure for T1D
JDRF Walk Team
#KoaKurefort1d
JDRF Children's Congress
2023

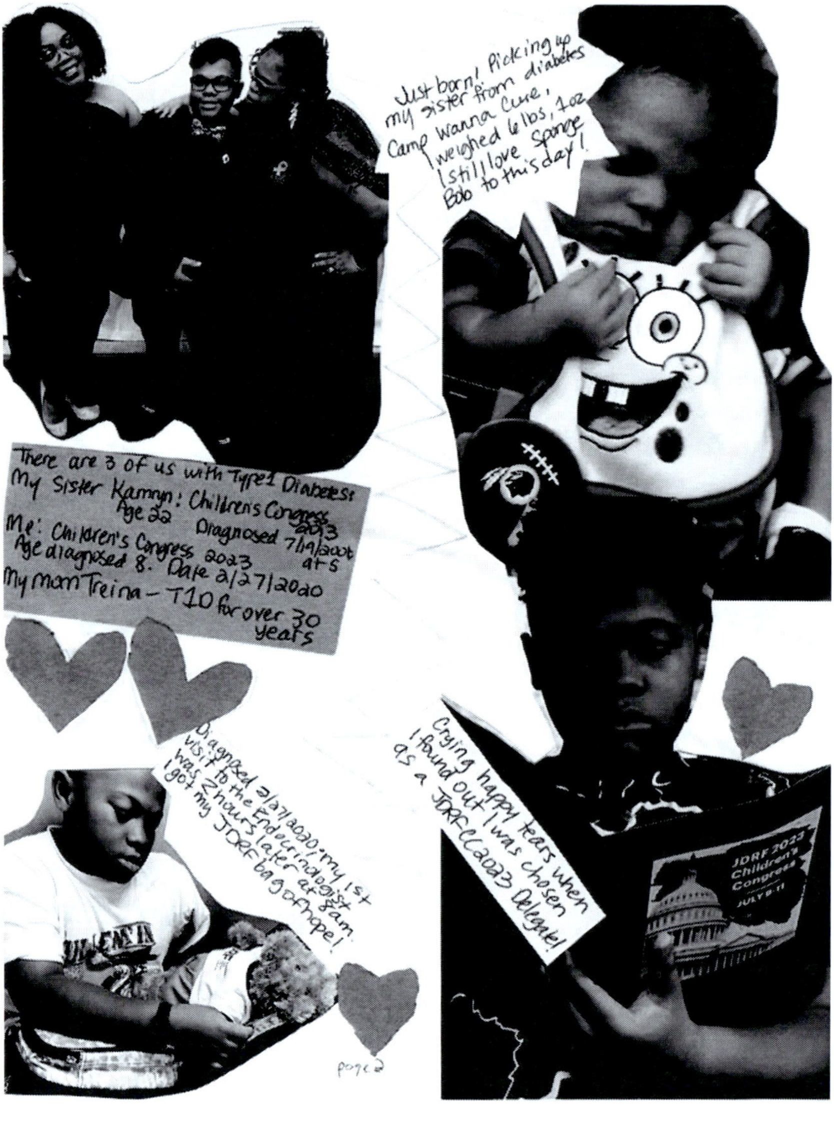
Just born! Picking up my sister from diabetes Camp Wanna Cure, I weighed 6 lbs, 7 oz. I still love Sponge Bob to this day!
There are 3 of us with Type1 Diabetes: My Sister Kamryn: Children's Congress 2013 Age 22 Diagnosed 7/19/2006 at 5
Me: Children's Congress 2023 Age diagnosed 8. Date 2/27/2020
My mom Treina – T1D for over 30 years
Diagnosed 2/27/2020, my 1st visit to the Endocrinologist was 2 hours later at 8am. I got my JDRF bag of hope!
Crying happy tears when I found out I was chosen as a JDRF CC 2023 Delegate!
JDRF 2023 Children's Congress JULY 9-11
page 2

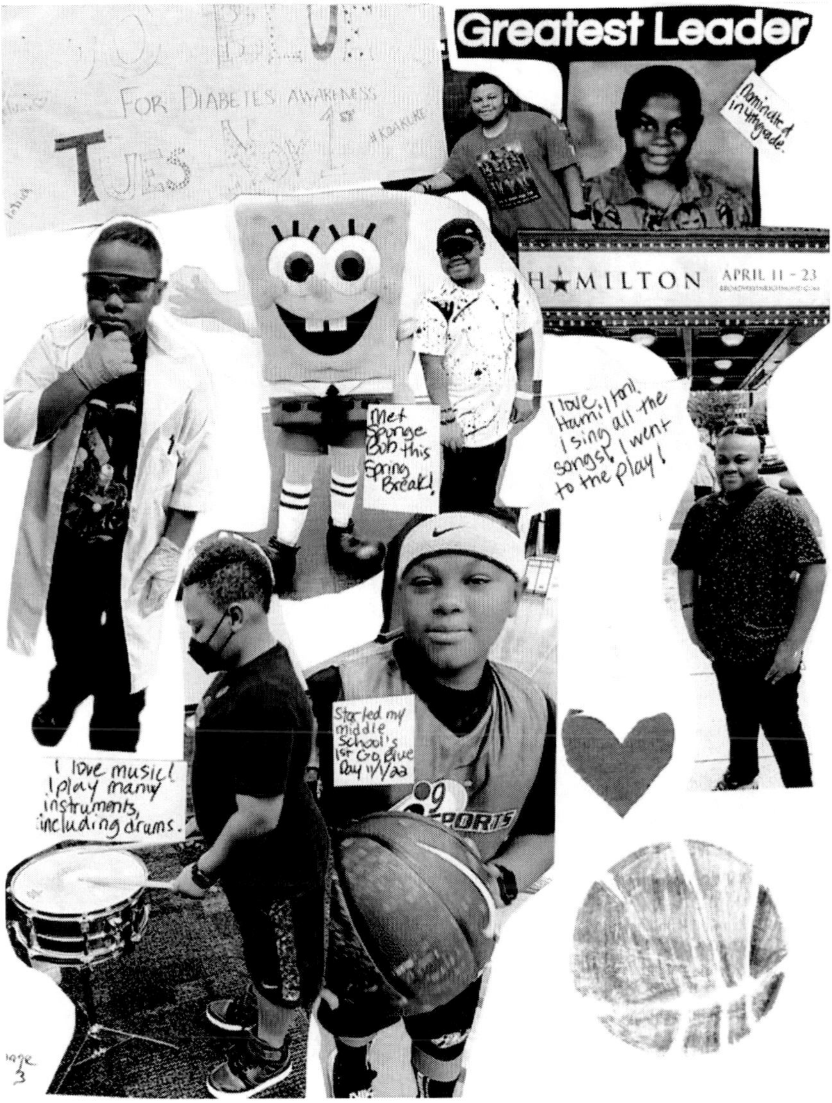
For Diabetes Awareness
Tues Nov 1st
Greatest Leader
HAMILTON APRIL 11 - 23
Met Sponge Bob this Spring Break!
I love Hamilton. I sing all the songs! I went to the play!
Started my middle School's 1st Go Blue Day 11/1/22
I love music! I play many instruments, including drums.

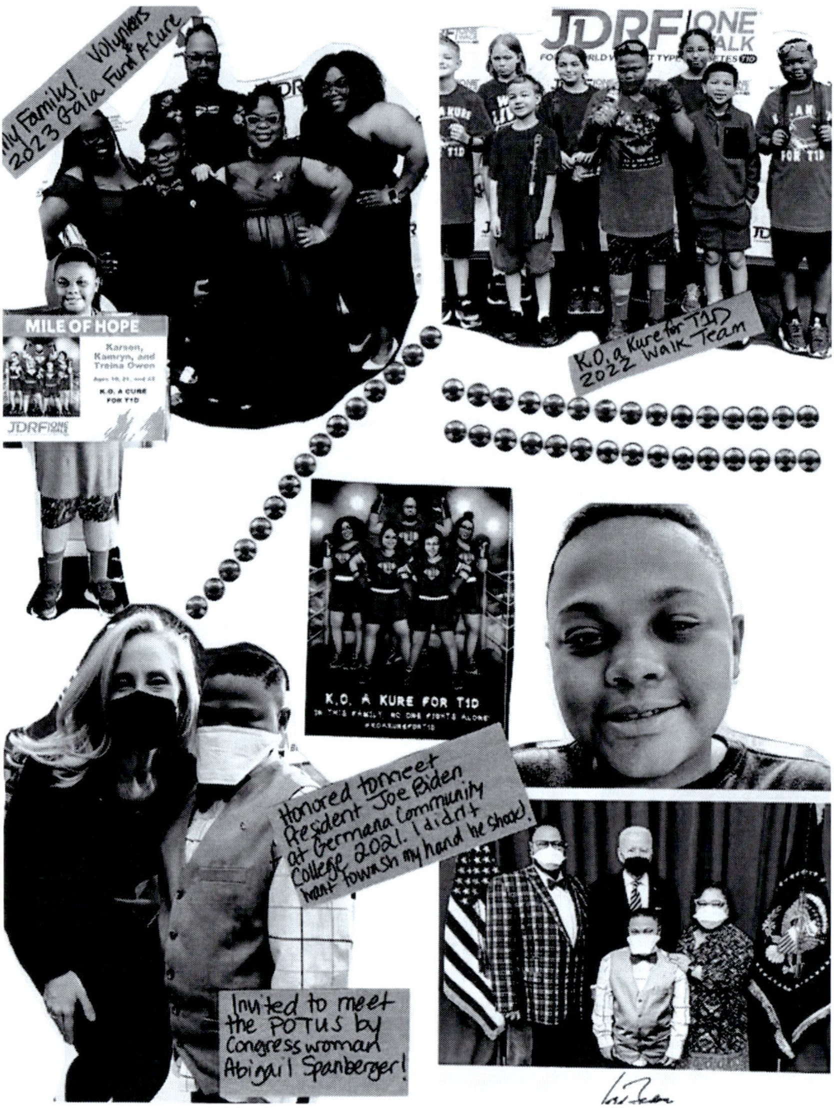
Family! Volunteers & 2023 Gala Fund A Cure
JDRF ONE WALK
MILE OF HOPE
Karsen, Kamryn, and Treina Owen
K.O. A CURE FOR T1D
JDRF ONE WALK
K.O. a Kure for T1D 2022 Walk Team
K.O. A KURE FOR T1D
IN THIS FAMILY, NO ONE FIGHTS ALONE
Honored to meet President Joe Biden at Germana Community College 2021. I didn't want to wash my hand he shook!
Invited to meet the POTUS by Congresswoman Abigail Spanberger!

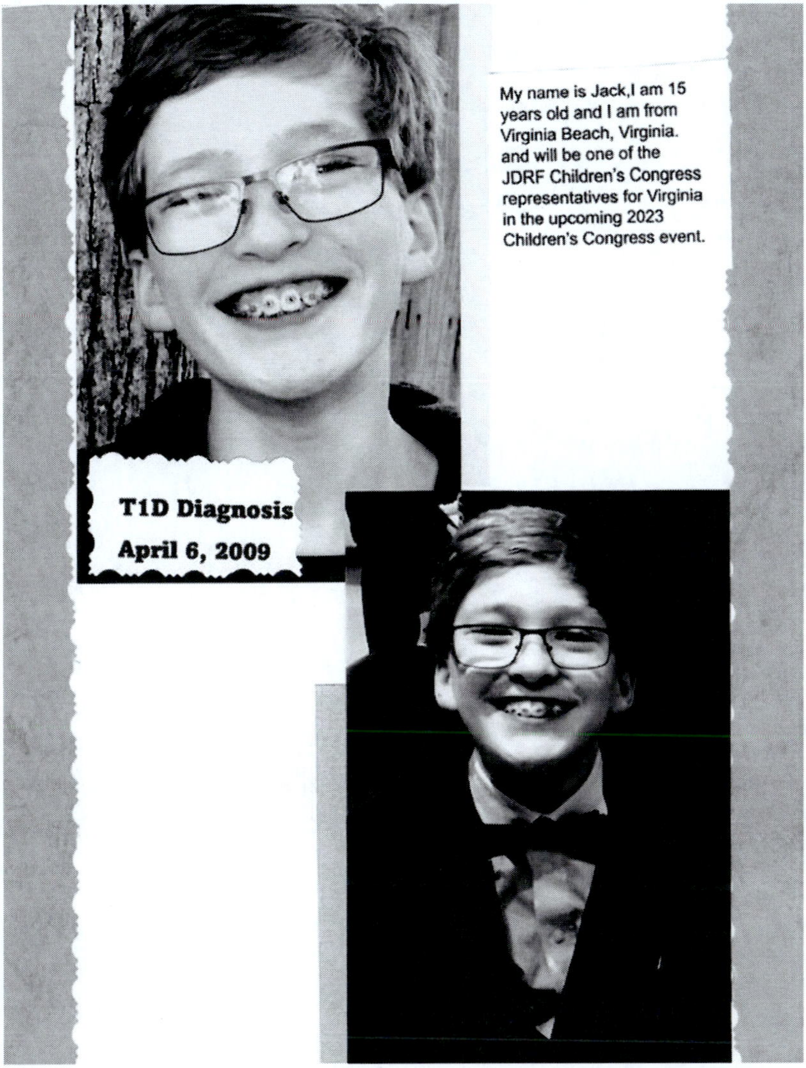
My name is Jack,I am 15 years old and I am from Virginia Beach, Virginia. and will be one of the JDRF Children's Congress representatives for Virginia in the upcoming 2023 Children's Congress event.
T1D Diagnosis
April 6, 2009

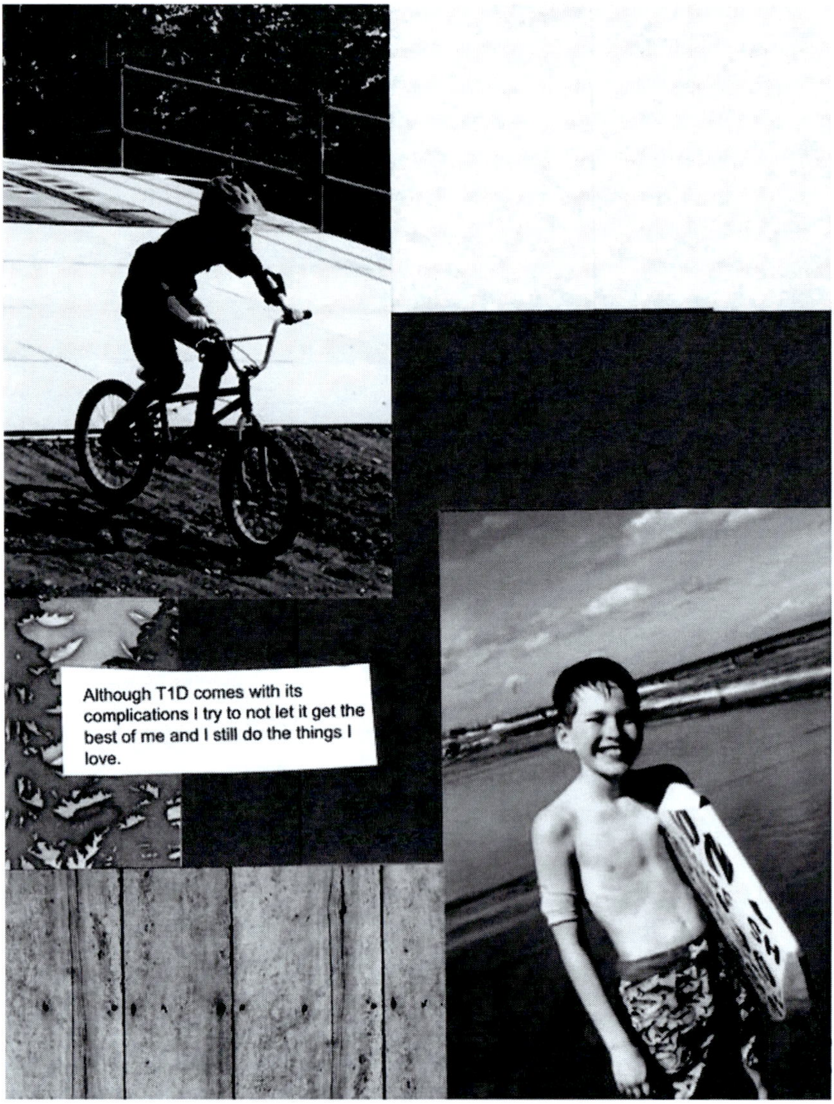
Although T1D comes with its complications I try to not let it get the best of me and I still do the things I love.

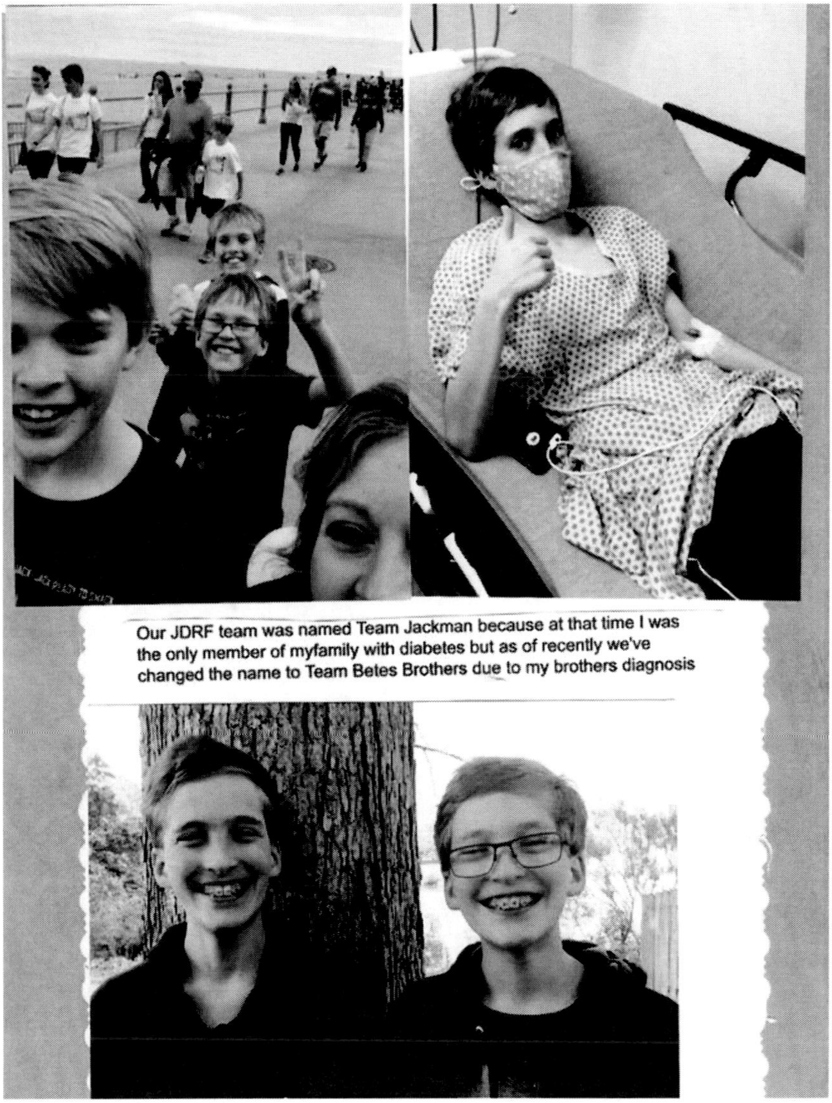
Our JDRF team was named Team Jackman because at that time I was
the only member of myfamily with diabetes but as of recently we've
changed the name to Team Betes Brothers due to my brothers diagnosis

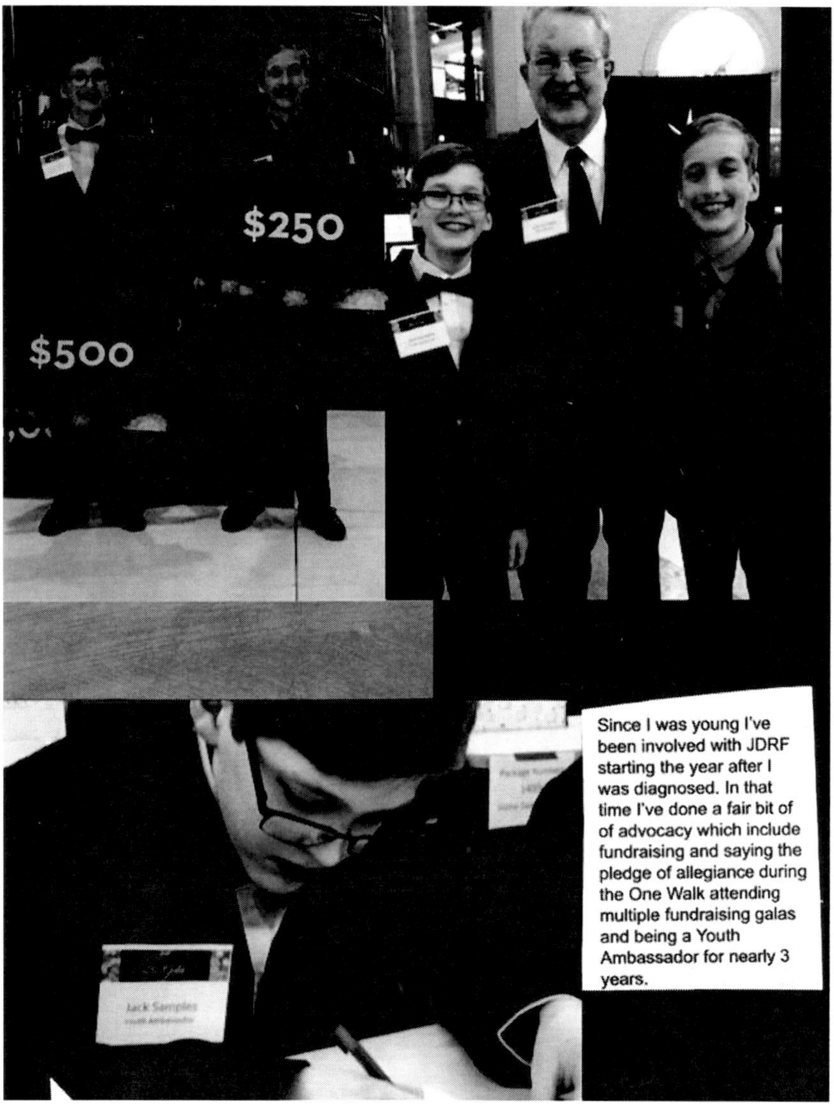
$250
$500
Since I was young I've been involved with JDRF starting the year after I was diagnosed. In that time I've done a fair bit of of advocacy which include fundraising and saying the pledge of allegiance during the One Walk attending multiple fundraising galas and being a Youth Ambassador for nearly 3 years.

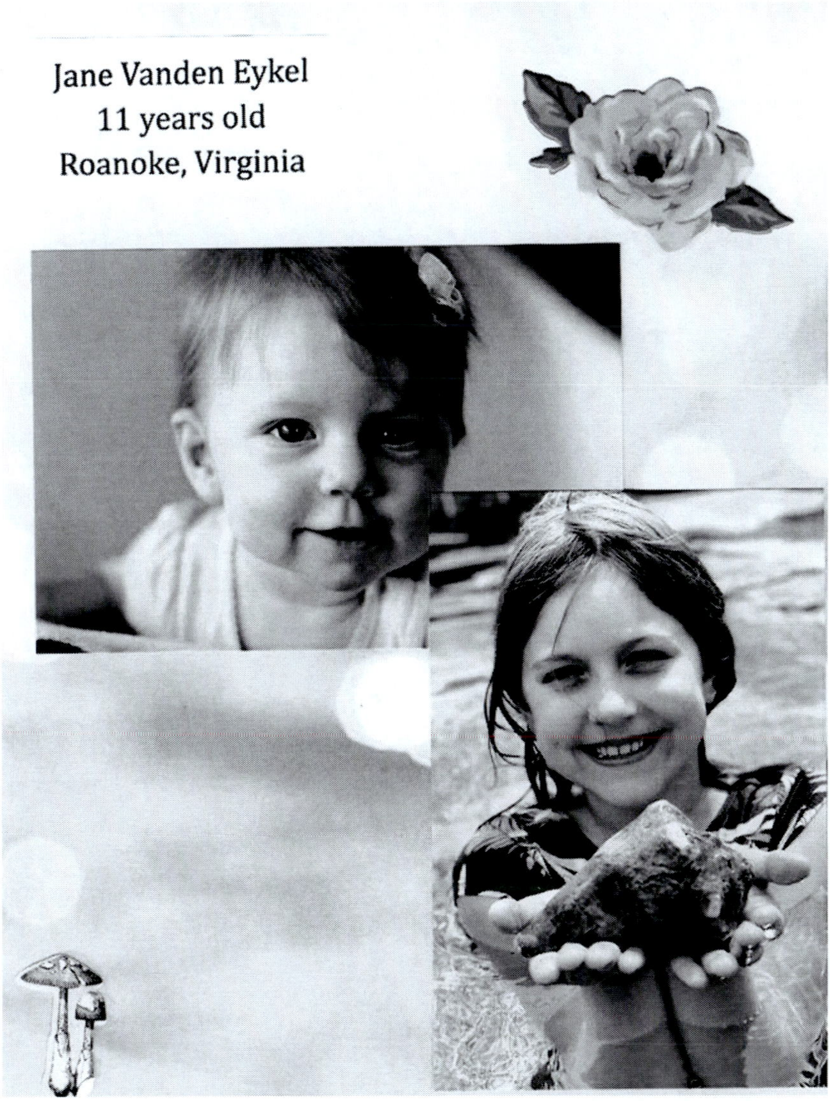
Jane Vanden Eykel
11 years old
Roanoke, Virginia

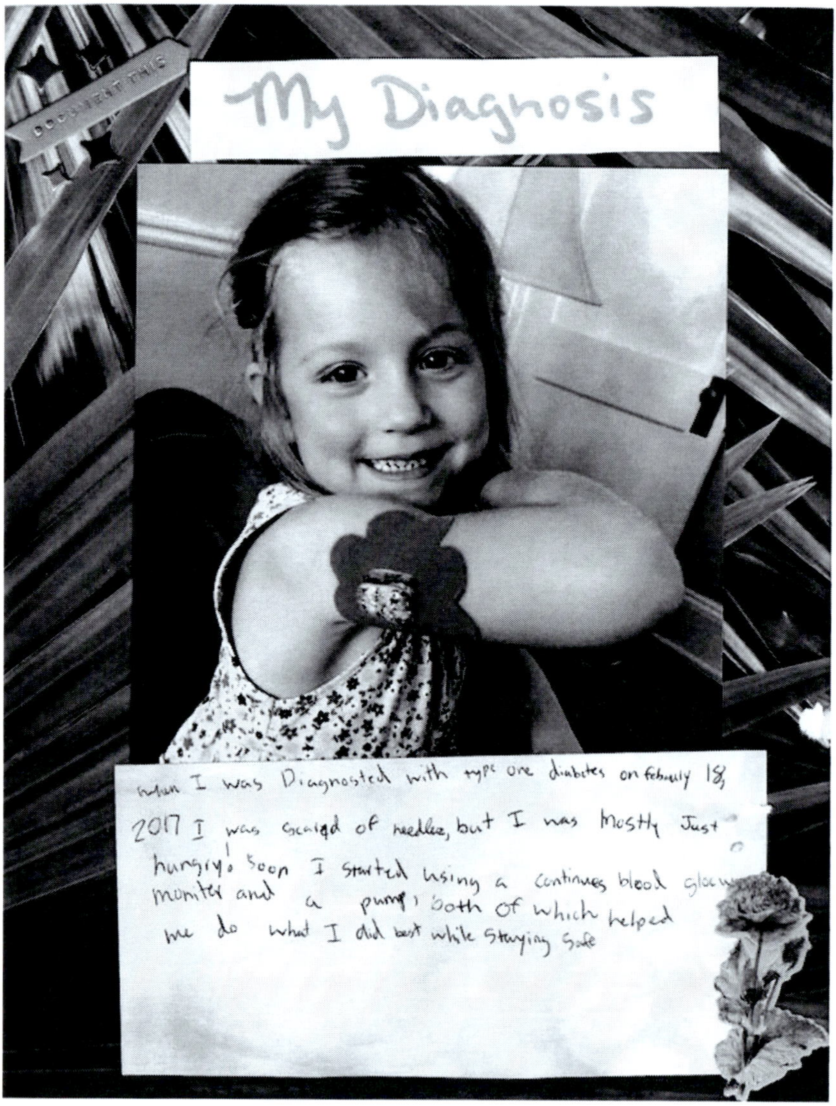
DOCUMENT THIS
My Diagnosis
when I was Diagnosted with type one diabetes on febuuly 18,
2017 I was scaired of needles, but I was mostly Just
hungry! Soon I started using a continues blood glocu
moniter and a pump, both of which helped
me do what I did best while staying safe

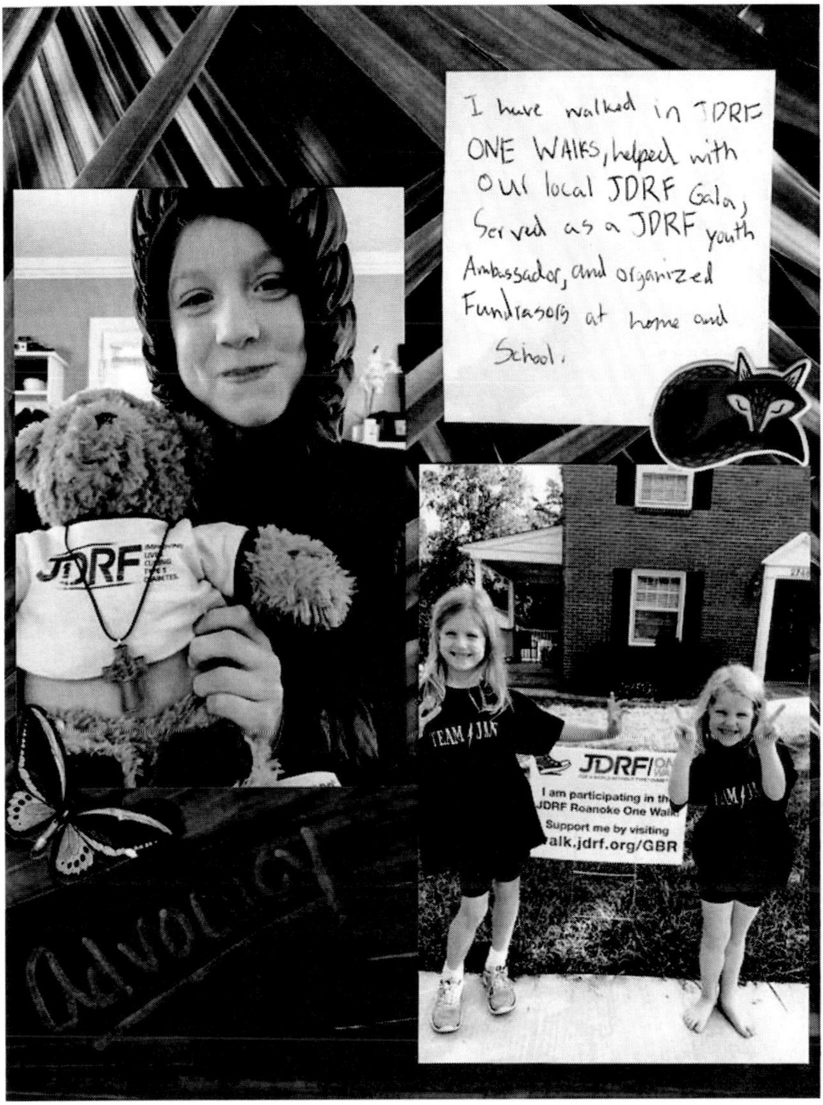
I have walked in JDRF ONE WALKS, helped with our local JDRF Gala, Served as a JDRF youth Ambassador, and organized Fundrasors at home and School.
JDRF
TEAM JAK
JDRF ONE WALK
I am participating in the JDRF Roanoke One Walk
Support me by visiting
walk.jdrf.org/GBR
Advocacy

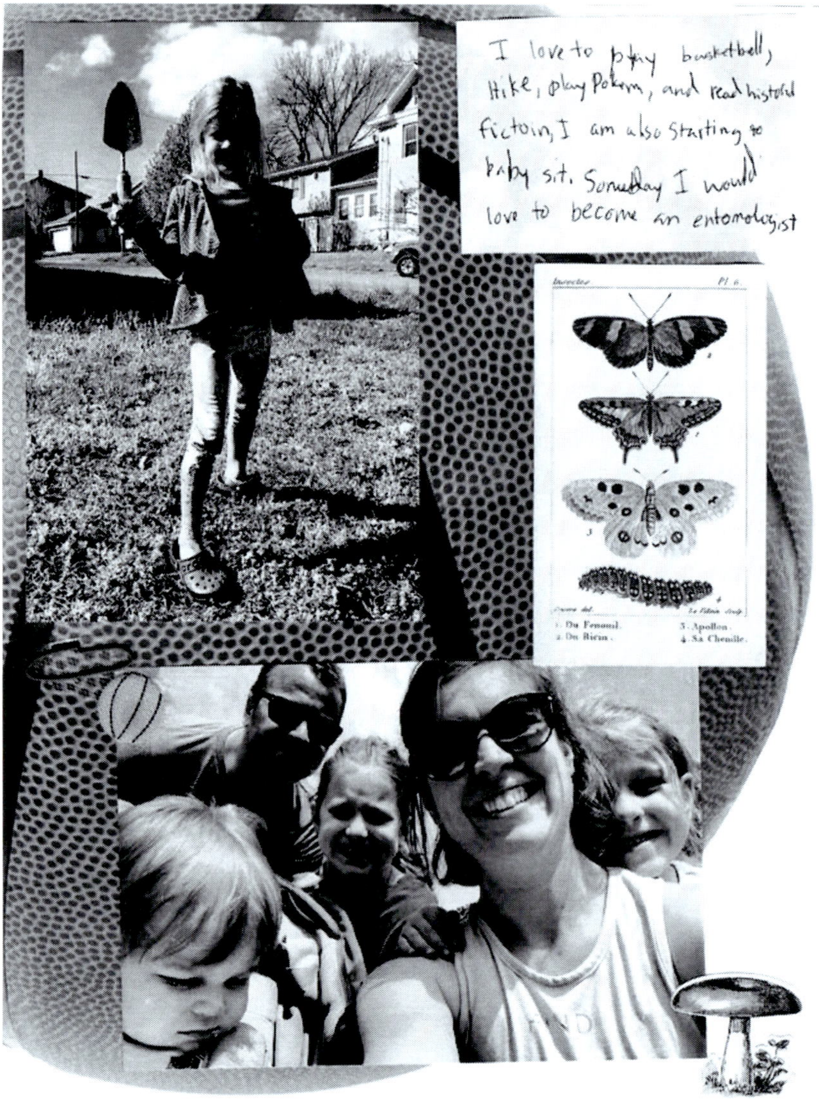
I love to play basketball,
Hike, play Pokem, and read histohl
fictoin, I am also Starting to
baby sit. Someday I would
love to become an entomologist
Pl. 6.
1. Du Fenouil.
2. Du Ricin.
3. Apollon.
4. Sa Chenille.

[Whereupon, at 11:39 a.m., the hearing was adjourned.]

## Chapter 2

# What Is Diabetes?*

## National Institute of Diabetes and Digestive and Kidney Diseases

Diabetes is a disease that occurs when your blood glucose, also called blood sugar, is too high. Glucose is your body's main source of energy. Your body can make glucose, but glucose also comes from the food you eat.

*Insulin* is a *hormone* made by the *pancreas* that helps glucose get into your cells to be used for energy. If you have diabetes, your body doesn't make enough—or any—insulin, or doesn't use insulin properly. Glucose then stays in your blood and doesn't reach your cells.

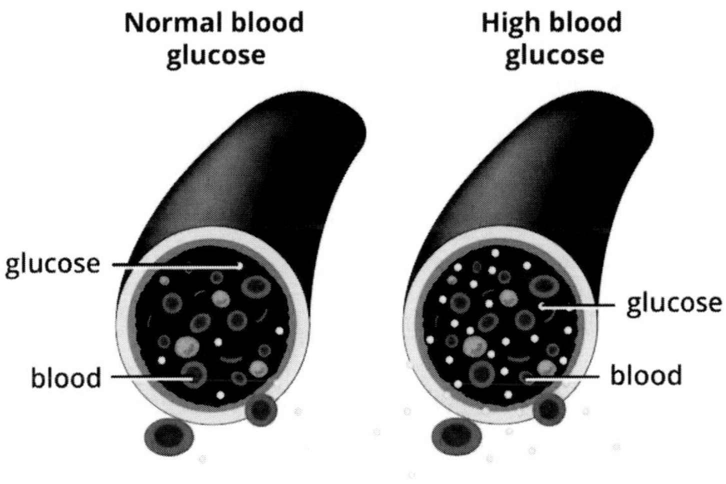


---

* This is an edited, reformatted and augmented version of National Institute of Diabetes and Digestive and Kidney Diseases Publication, Last Reviewed April 2023.

In: Comprehensive Diabetes Care
Editor: Joseph S. Green
ISBN: 979-8-89530-772-4

Diabetes raises the risk for damage to the eyes, kidneys, nerves, and heart. Diabetes is also linked to some types of cancer. Taking steps to prevent or manage diabetes may lower your risk of developing diabetes health problems.

Diabetes is a disease that occurs when your blood glucose, also called blood sugar, is too high.

## What Are the Different Types of Diabetes?

The most common types of diabetes are type 1, type 2, and gestational diabetes.

### Type 1 Diabetes

If you have type 1 diabetes, your body makes little or no insulin. Your immune system attacks and destroys the cells in your pancreas that make insulin. Type 1 diabetes is usually diagnosed in children and young adults, although it can appear at any age. People with type 1 diabetes need to take insulin every day to stay alive.

### Type 2 Diabetes

If you have type 2 diabetes, the cells in your body don't use insulin properly. The pancreas may be making insulin but is not making enough insulin to keep your blood glucose level in the normal range. Type 2 diabetes is the most common type of diabetes. You are more likely to develop type 2 diabetes if you have risk factors, such as overweight or obesity, and a family history of the disease. You can develop type 2 diabetes at any age, even during childhood.

You can help delay or prevent type 2 diabetes by knowing the risk factors and taking steps toward a healthier lifestyle, such as losing weight or preventing weight gain.

## Gestational Diabetes

Gestational diabetes is a type of diabetes that develops during pregnancy. Most of the time, this type of diabetes goes away after the baby is born. However, if you've had gestational diabetes, you have a higher chance of developing type 2 diabetes later in life. Sometimes diabetes diagnosed during pregnancy is type 2 diabetes.

## Prediabetes

People with prediabetes have blood glucose levels that are higher than normal but not high enough to be diagnosed with type 2 diabetes. If you have prediabetes, you have a higher risk of developing type 2 diabetes in the future. You also have a higher risk for heart disease than people with normal glucose levels.

## Other Types of Diabetes

A less common type of diabetes, called monogenic diabetes, is caused by a change in a single gene. Diabetes can also come from having surgery to remove the pancreas, or from damage to the pancreas due to conditions such as cystic fibrosis *NIH external link* or pancreatitis.

## How Common Are Diabetes and Prediabetes?

More than 133 million Americans have diabetes or prediabetes [1].

As of 2019, 37.3 million people—or 11.3% of the U.S. population—had diabetes [1]. More than 1 in 4 people over the age of 65 had diabetes. Nearly 1 in 4 adults with diabetes didn't know they had the disease [2].

About 90% to 95% of diabetes cases are type 2 diabetes [3]. In 2019, 96 million adults—38% of U.S. adults—had prediabetes [4].

## What Other Health Problems Can People with Diabetes Develop?

Over time, high blood glucose can damage your heart, kidneys, feet, and eyes. If you have diabetes, you can take steps to lower your chances of developing diabetes health problems by taking steps to improve your health and learning how to manage the disease. Managing your blood glucose, blood pressure, and cholesterol levels can help prevent future health problems.

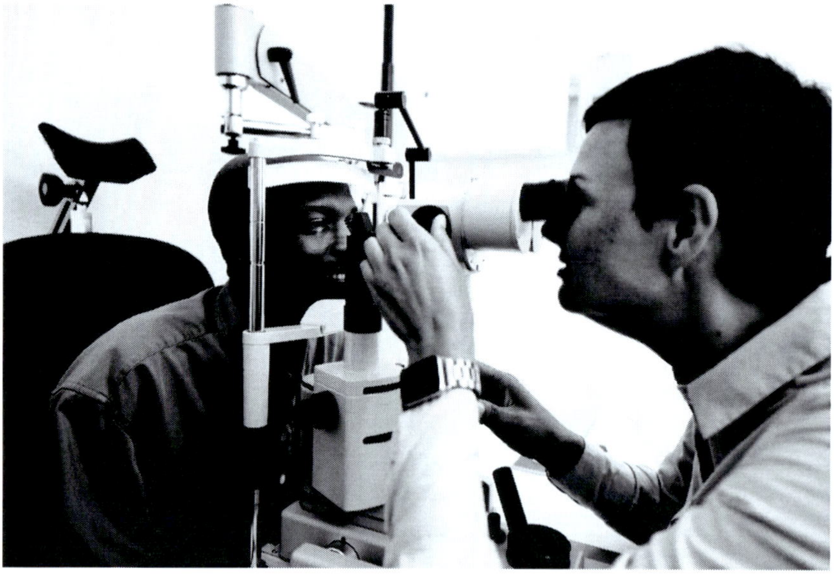

Managing your blood glucose levels can help prevent future health problems, such as damage to your eyes.

## References


[1] National diabetes statistics report, 2022. Centers for Disease Control and Prevention. Updated January 18, 2022. Accessed August 4, 2022. www.cdc.gov/diabetes/php/data-research/ External link.

[2] Prevalence of both diagnosed and undiagnosed diabetes. National diabetes statistics report, 2022. Centers for Disease Control and Prevention. Updated September 30, 2022. Accessed November 1, 2022. www.cdc.gov/diabetes/php/data-research/ External link.

[3] Methods. National diabetes statistics report, 2022. Centers for Disease Control and Prevention. Updated September 30, 2022. Accessed November 1, 2022. www.cdc.gov/diabetes/php/data-research/methods.html External link.

[4] Prevalence of prediabetes among adults. National diabetes statistics report, 2022. Centers for Disease Control and Prevention. Updated September 30, 2022. Accessed November 1, 2022. www.cdc.gov/diabetes/php/data-research/ External link.

Chapter 3

# Type 1 Diabetes*

## National Institute of Diabetes and Digestive and Kidney Diseases

### What Is Type 1 Diabetes?

Diabetes occurs when your blood glucose, also called blood sugar, is too high. Blood glucose is your main source of energy and comes mainly from the food you eat. Insulin, a hormone made by the pancreas, helps the glucose in your blood get into your cells to be used for energy. Another hormone, glucagon, works with insulin to control blood glucose levels.

In most people with type 1 diabetes, the body's immune system, which normally fights infection, attacks and destroys the cells in the pancreas that make insulin. As a result, your pancreas stops making insulin. Without insulin, glucose can't get into your cells and your blood glucose rises above normal. People with type 1 diabetes need to take insulin every day to stay alive.

### Who Is More Likely to Develop Type 1 Diabetes?

Type 1 diabetes typically occurs in children and young adults, although it can appear at any age. Having a parent or sibling with the disease may increase your chance of developing type 1 diabetes. In the United States, about 5 percent of people with diabetes have type 1 [1].

---

* This is an edited, reformatted and augmented version of National Institute of Diabetes and Digestive and Kidney Diseases Publication.

In: Comprehensive Diabetes Care
Editor: Joseph S. Green
ISBN: 979-8-89530-772-4

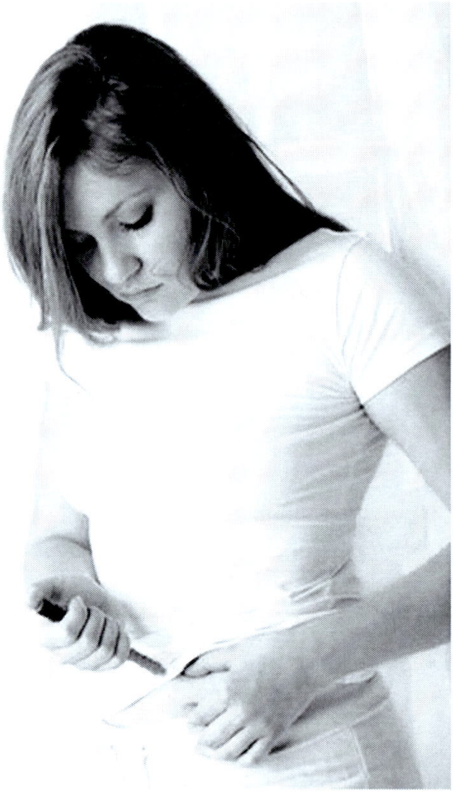

People with type 1 diabetes need to take insulin every day.

## What Are The Symptoms of Type 1 Diabetes?

Symptoms of type 1 diabetes are serious and usually happen quickly, over a few days to weeks. Symptoms can include

- increased thirst and urination
- increased hunger
- blurred vision
- fatigue
- unexplained weight loss

Sometimes the first symptoms of type 1 diabetes are signs of a life-threatening condition called diabetic ketoacidosis (DKA) *NIH external link.* Some symptoms of DKA include

- breath that smells fruity
- dry or flushed skin
- nausea or vomiting
- stomach pain
- trouble breathing
- trouble paying attention or feeling confused

DKA is serious and dangerous. If you or your child have symptoms of DKA, contact your health care professional right away, or go to the nearest hospital emergency room.

## What Causes Type 1 Diabetes?

Experts think type 1 diabetes is caused by genes and factors in the environment, such as viruses, that might trigger the disease. Researchers are working to pinpoint the causes of type 1 diabetes through studies such as TrialNet External link.

## How Do Health Care Professionals Diagnose Type 1 Diabetes?

Health care professionals usually test people for type 1 diabetes if they have clear-cut diabetes symptoms. Health care professionals most often use the random plasma glucose (RPG) test to diagnose type 1 diabetes. This blood test measures your blood glucose level at a single point in time. Sometimes health professionals also use the A1C blood test to find out how long someone has had high blood glucose.

Even though these tests can confirm that you have diabetes, they can't identify what type you have. Treatment depends on the type of diabetes, so knowing whether you have type 1 or type 2 is important.

To find out if your diabetes is type 1, your health care professional may test your blood for certain autoantibodies. Autoantibodies are antibodies that attack your healthy tissues and cells by mistake. The presence of certain types of autoantibodies is common in type 1 but not in type 2 diabetes.

Because type 1 diabetes can run in families, your health care professional can test your family members for autoantibodies. Type 1 diabetes TrialNet, an international research network, also offers autoantibody testing to family members External link of people diagnosed with the disease. The presence of autoantibodies, even without diabetes symptoms, means the family member is more likely to develop type 1 diabetes. If you have a brother or sister, child, or parent with type 1 diabetes, you may want to get an autoantibody test. People age 20 or younger who have a cousin, aunt, uncle, niece, nephew, grandparent, or half-sibling with type 1 diabetes also may want to get tested.

## What Medicines Do I Need to Treat My Type 1 Diabetes?

If you have type 1 diabetes, you must take insulin because your body no longer makes this hormone. Different types of insulin start to work at different speeds, and the effects of each last a different length of time. You may need to use more than one type. You can take insulin a number of ways. Common options include a needle and syringe, insulin pen, or insulin pump.

Some people who have trouble reaching their blood glucose targets with insulin alone also might need to take another type of diabetes medicine that works with insulin, such as pramlintide *NIH external link*. Pramlintide, given by injection, helps keep blood glucose levels from going too high after eating. Few people with type 1 diabetes take pramlintide, however. The NIH has recently funded a large research study to test use of pramlintide along with insulin and glucagon in people with type 1 diabetes. Another diabetes medicine, metformin, may help decrease the amount of insulin you need to take, but more studies are needed to confirm this. Reseachers are also studying other diabetes pills that people with type 1 diabetes might take along with insulin.

Hypoglycemia, or low blood sugar, can occur if you take insulin but don't match your dose with your food or physical activity. Severe hypoglycemia can be dangerous and needs to be treated right away. Learn more about hypoglycemia and how to prevent or treat it.

## How Else Can I Manage Type 1 Diabetes?

Along with insulin and any other medicines you use, you can manage your diabetes by taking care of yourself each day. Following your diabetes meal plan, being physically active, and checking your blood glucose often are some of the ways you can take care of yourself. Work with your health care team to come up with a diabetes care plan that works for you. If you are planning a pregnancy with diabetes, try to get your blood glucose levels in your target range before you get pregnant.

## Do I Have Other Treatment Options for My Type 1 Diabetes?

The National Institute of Diabetes and Digestive and Kidney Diseases (NIDDK) has played an important role in developing "artificial pancreas" technology. An artificial pancreas replaces manual blood glucose testing and the use of insulin shots. A single system monitors blood glucose levels around the clock and provides insulin or a combination of insulin and glucagon automatically. The system can also be monitored remotely, for example by parents or medical staff.

In 2016, the U.S. Food and Drug Administration approved a type of artificial pancreas system called a hybrid closed-loop system. This system tests your glucose level every 5 minutes throughout the day and night through a continuous glucose monitor, and automatically gives you the right amount of basal insulin, a long-acting insulin, through a separate insulin pump. You still need to manually adjust the amount of insulin the pump delivers at mealtimes and when you need a correction dose. You also will need to test your blood with a glucose meter several times a day. Talk with your health care provider about whether this system might be right for you.

The illustration below shows the parts of a type of artificial pancreas system.

An artificial pancreas system uses a continuous glucose monitor, an insulin pump, and a control algorithm to give you the right amount of basal insulin.

The continuous glucose monitor sends information through a software program called a control algorithm. Based on your glucose level, the algorithm tells the insulin pump how much insulin to deliver. The software program could be installed on the pump or another device such as a cell phone or computer.

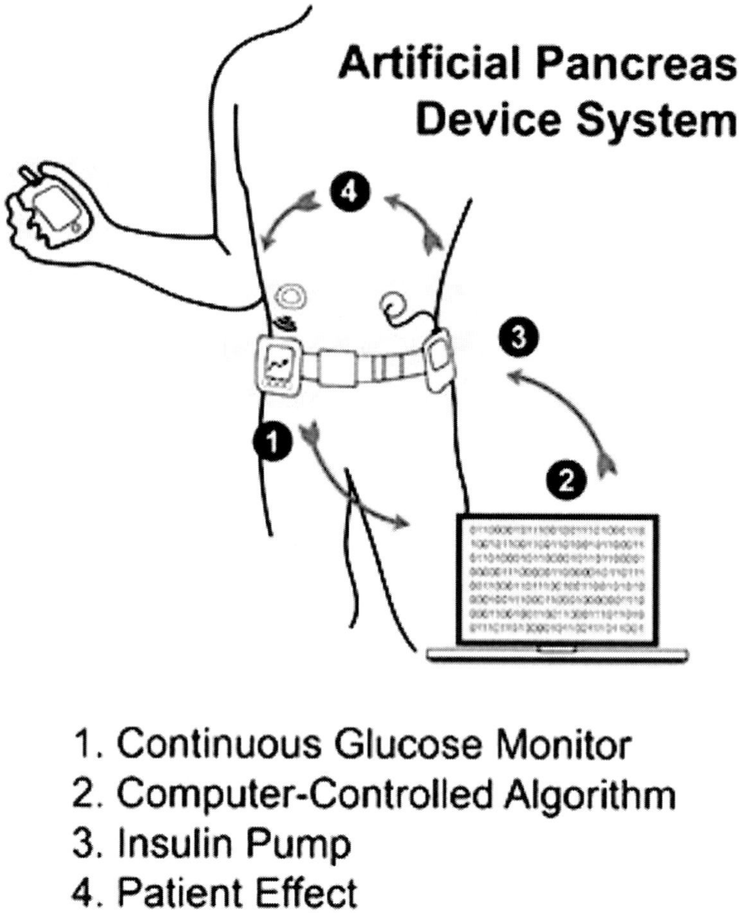


Starting in late 2016 and early 2017, the NIDDK has funded several important studies NIH external link on different types of artificial pancreas devices to better help people with type 1 diabetes manage their disease. The devices may also help people with type 2 diabetes and gestational diabetes.

NIDDK also supported research into pancreatic islet transplantation—a treatment for type 1 diabetes in people who struggle to manage their blood glucose levels. Pancreatic islets are clusters of cells in the pancreas that make the hormone insulin. In type 1 diabetes, the body's immune system attacks these cells. A pancreatic islet transplant replaces destroyed islets with new islets from a deceased donor. The new islets make and release insulin.

## What Health Problems Can People with Type 1 Diabetes Develop?

Over time, high blood glucose leads to problems such as

- heart disease
- stroke
- kidney disease
- eye problems
- dental disease
- nerve damage
- foot problems
- depression
- sleep apnea

If you have type 1 diabetes, you can help prevent or delay the health problems of diabetes by managing your blood glucose, blood pressure, and cholesterol, and following your self-care plan.

## Can I Lower My Chance of Developing Type 1 Diabetes?

At this time, type 1 diabetes can't be prevented. However, through studies such as TrialNet, researchers are working to identify possible ways to prevent or slow down the disease.

## Reference

[1] Centers for Disease Control and Prevention. National diabetes statistics report, 2017. Centers for Disease Control and Prevention website. www.cdc.gov/diabetes/pdfs/data/statistics/national-diabetes-statistics-report.pdf External link (PDF, 1.3 MB) . Updated July, 18 2017. Accessed August 1, 2017.

## Chapter 4

# Type 2 Diabetes*

## National Institute of Diabetes and Digestive and Kidney Diseases

### What Is Type 2 Diabetes?

Type 2 diabetes, the most common type of diabetes, is a disease that occurs when your blood glucose, also called blood sugar, is too high. Blood glucose is your main source of energy and comes mainly from the food you eat. Insulin, a hormone made by the pancreas, helps glucose get into your cells to be used for energy. In type 2 diabetes, your body doesn't make enough insulin or doesn't use insulin well. Too much glucose then stays in your blood, and not enough reaches your cells.

The good news is that you can take steps to prevent or delay the development of type 2 diabetes.

### Who Is More Likely to Develop Type 2 Diabetes?

You can develop type 2 diabetes at any age, even during childhood. However, type 2 diabetes occurs most often in middle-aged and older people. You are more likely to develop type 2 diabetes if you are age 45 or older, have a family history of diabetes, or are overweight or have obesity. Diabetes is more

* This is an edited, reformatted and augmented version of National Institute of Diabetes and Digestive and Kidney Diseases Publication.

In: Comprehensive Diabetes Care
Editor: Joseph S. Green
ISBN: 979-8-89530-772-4

common in people who are African American, Hispanic/Latino, American Indian, Asian American, or Pacific Islander.

Physical inactivity and certain health problems such as high blood pressure affect your chances of developing type 2 diabetes. You are also more likely to develop type 2 diabetes if you have prediabetes or had gestational diabetes when you were pregnant. Learn more about risk factors for type 2 diabetes.

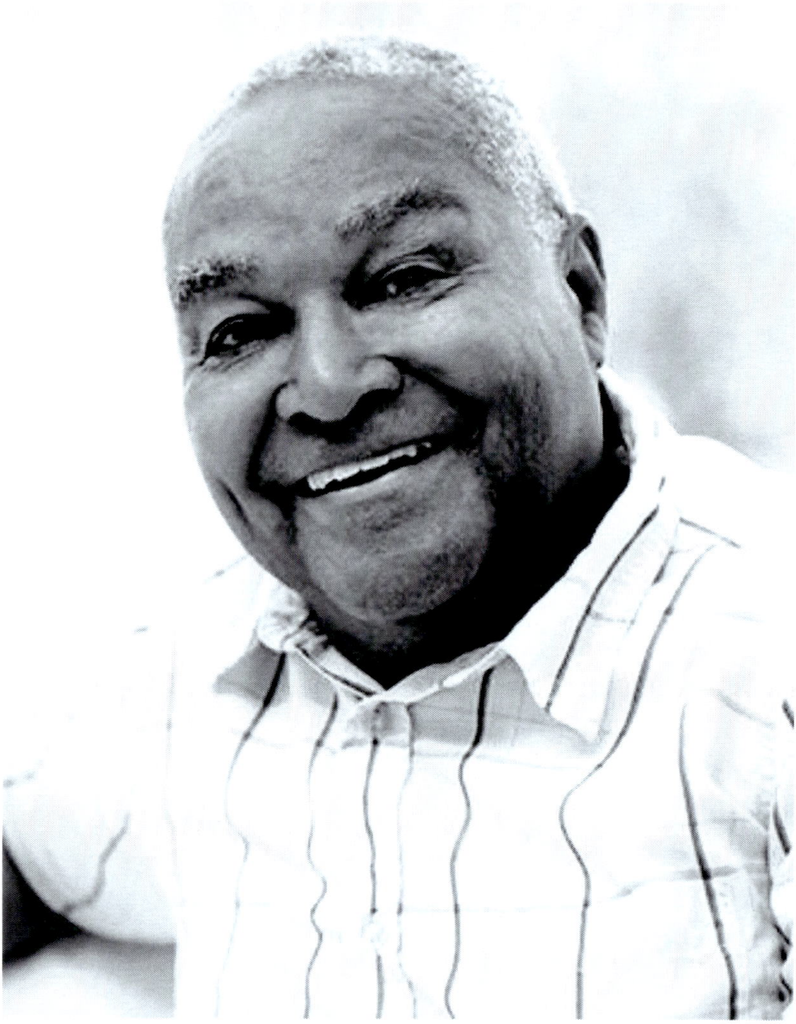

Type 2 diabetes occurs most often in middle-aged and older people.

## What Are the Symptoms of Diabetes?

Symptoms of diabetes include

- increased thirst and urination
- increased hunger
- feeling tired
- blurred vision
- numbness or tingling in the feet or hands
- sores that do not heal
- unexplained weight loss

Symptoms of type 2 diabetes often develop slowly—over the course of several years—and can be so mild that you might not even notice them. Many people have no symptoms. Some people do not find out they have the disease until they have diabetes-related health problems, such as blurred vision or heart disease.

## What Causes Type 2 Diabetes?

Type 2 diabetes is caused by several factors, including

- overweight and obesity
- not being physically active
- insulin resistance
- genes

Learn more about the causes of type 2 diabetes.

## How Do Health Care Professionals Diagnose Type 2 Diabetes?

Your health care professional can diagnose type 2 diabetes based on blood tests. Learn more about blood tests for diabetes and what the results mean.

## How Can I Manage My Type 2 Diabetes?

Managing your blood glucose, blood pressure, and cholesterol, and quitting smoking if you smoke, are important ways to manage your type 2 diabetes. Lifestyle changes that include planning healthy meals, limiting calories if you are overweight, and being physically active are also part of managing your diabetes. So is taking any prescribed medicines. Work with your health care team to create a diabetes care plan that works for you.

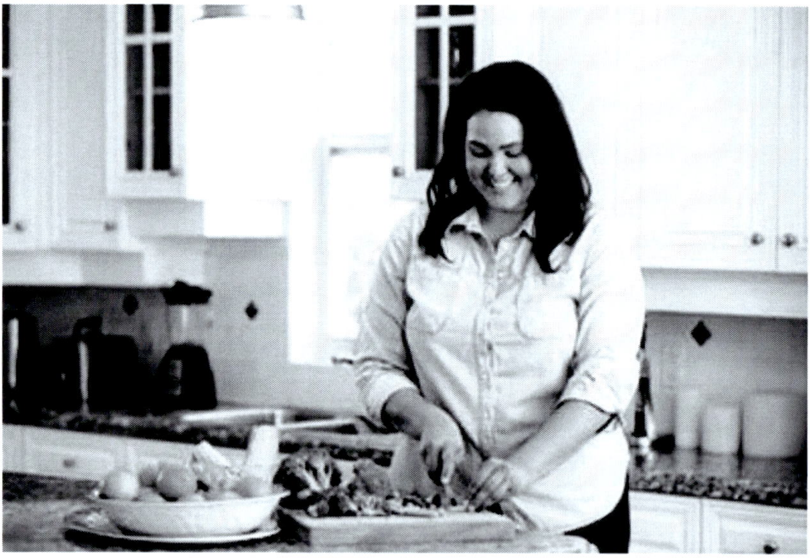

Following your meal plan helps you manage your diabetes.

## What Medicines Do I Need to Treat My Type 2 Diabetes?

Along with following your diabetes care plan, you may need diabetes medicines, which may include pills or medicines you inject under your skin, such as insulin. Over time, you may need more than one diabetes medicine to manage your blood glucose. Even if you don't take insulin, you may need it at special times, such as during pregnancy or if you are in the hospital. You also may need medicines for high blood pressure, high cholesterol, or other conditions.

Learn more about medicines, insulin, and other diabetes treatments.

## What Health Problems Can People with Diabetes Develop?

Following a good diabetes care plan can help protect against many diabetes-related health problems. However, if not managed, diabetes can lead to problems such as

- heart disease and stroke
- nerve damage
- kidney disease
- foot problems
- eye disease
- gum disease and other dental problems
- sexual and bladder problems

Many people with type 2 diabetes also have nonalcoholic fatty liver disease (NAFLD). Losing weight if you are overweight or have obesity can improve NAFLD. Diabetes is also linked to other health problems such as sleep apnea, depression, some types of cancer, and dementia *NIH external link*.

You can take steps to lower your chances of developing these diabetes-related health problems.

## How Can I Lower My Chances of Developing Type 2 Diabetes?

Research such as the Diabetes Prevention Program External link, sponsored by the National Institutes of Health, has shown that you can take steps to reduce your chances of developing type 2 diabetes if you have risk factors for the disease. Here are some things you can do to lower your risk:

- Lose weight if you are overweight, and keep it off. You may be able to prevent or delay diabetes by losing 5 to 7 percent of your current weight [1]. For instance, if you weigh 200 pounds, your goal would be to lose about 10 to 14 pounds.

Diabetes Risk Management Calculator
Losing 5% to 7% of your body weight may reduce your risk of diabetes.†
Heightin feet

Weightin pounds

† For adults 20 and older at high risk of developing type 2 diabetes Back to content

Supported by a study from

- *Move more.* Get at least 30 minutes of physical activity, such as walking, at least 5 days a week. If you have not been active, talk with your health care professional about which activities are best. Start slowly and build up to your goal.
- *Eat healthy foods.* Eat smaller portions to reduce the amount of calories you eat each day and help you lose weight. Choosing foods with less fat is another way to reduce calories. Drink water instead of sweetened beverages.

Ask your health care team what other changes you can make to prevent or delay type 2 diabetes.

Most often, your best chance for preventing type 2 diabetes is to make lifestyle changes that work for you long term. Get started with Your Game Plan to Prevent Type 2 Diabetes.

## Reference

[1] Diabetes Prevention Program Research Group. Long-term effects of lifestyle intervention or metformin on diabetes development and microvascular complications over 15-year follow-up: the Diabetes Prevention Program Outcomes Study. *The Lancet Diabetes & Endocrinology*. 2015;3(11):866–875. You can find more information about this study on the Diabetes Prevention Program Outcomes Study website.

## Chapter 5

# Healthy Living with Diabetes*


## National Institute of Diabetes and Digestive and Kidney Diseases


Healthy living is a way to manage diabetes. To have a healthy lifestyle, take steps now to plan healthy meals and snacks, do physical activities, get enough sleep, and quit smoking or using tobacco products.

Healthy living may help keep your body's blood pressure, cholesterol, and blood glucose level, also called blood sugar level, in the range your primary health care professional recommends. Your primary health care professional may be a doctor, a physician assistant, or a nurse practitioner. Healthy living may also help prevent or delay health problems from diabetes that can affect your heart, kidneys, eyes, brain, and other parts of your body.

Making lifestyle changes can be hard, but starting with small changes and building from there may benefit your health. You may want to get help from family, loved ones, friends, and other trusted people in your community. You can also get information from your health care professionals.

## How Can I Plan What to Eat or Drink When I Have Diabetes?

What you choose to eat, how much you eat, and when you eat are parts of a meal plan. Having healthy foods and drinks can help keep your blood glucose, blood pressure, and cholesterol levels in the ranges your health care professional recommends. If you have overweight or obesity, a healthy meal

* This is an edited, reformatted and augmented version of National Institute of Diabetes and Digestive and Kidney Diseases Publication.


In: Comprehensive Diabetes Care
Editor: Joseph S. Green
ISBN: 979-8-89530-772-4

plan—along with regular physical activity, getting enough sleep, and other healthy behaviors—may help you reach and maintain a healthy weight. In some cases, health care professionals may also recommend diabetes medicines that may help you lose weight, or weight-loss surgery, also called metabolic and bariatric surgery.

## Choose Healthy Foods and Drinks

There is no right or wrong way to choose healthy foods and drinks that may help manage your diabetes. Healthy meal plans for people who have diabetes may include

- dairy or plant-based dairy products External link
- fruits External link
- nonstarchy vegetables External link
- protein foods External link
- whole grains External link

Try to choose foods that include nutrients such as vitamins, calcium NIH external link, fiber NIH external link, and healthy fats External link. Also try to choose drinks with little or no added sugar External link, such as tap or bottled water, low-fat or non-fat milk, and unsweetened tea, coffee, or sparkling water.

Try to plan meals and snacks that have fewer

- foods high in saturated fat NIH external link
- foods high in sodium, a mineral found in salt External link
- sugary foods External link, such as cookies and cakes, and sweet drinks, such as soda, juice, flavored coffee, and sports drinks

Your body turns carbohydrates NIH external link, or carbs, from food into glucose, which can raise your blood glucose level. Some fruits, beans, and starchy vegetables—such as potatoes and corn—have more carbs than other foods. Keep carbs in mind when planning your meals.

You should also limit how much alcohol External link you drink. If you take insulin or certain diabetes medicines, drinking alcohol can make your blood glucose level drop too low, which is called hypoglycemia. If you do drink alcohol, be sure to eat food when you drink and remember to check your blood glucose level after drinking. Talk with your health care team about your alcohol-drinking habits.

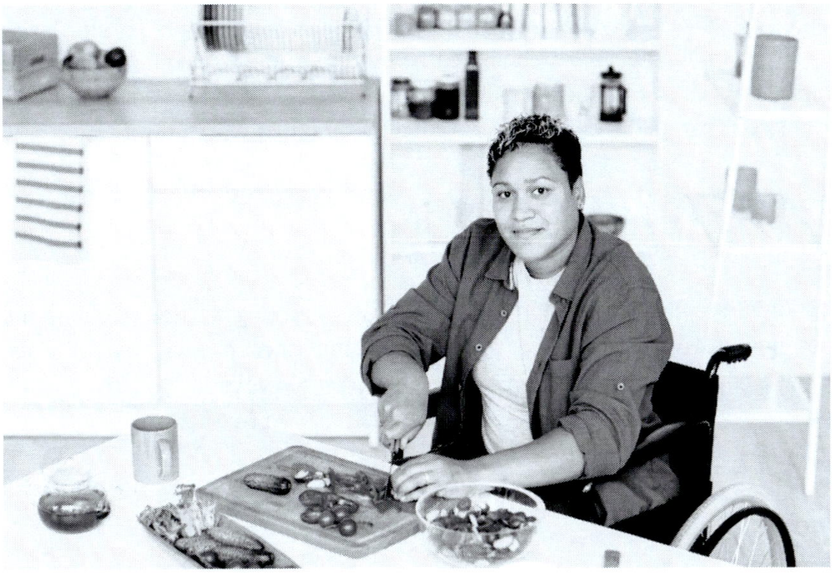

Try to choose foods that include nutrients such as vitamins, calcium, fiber, and healthy fats.

## Find the Best Times to Eat or Drink

Talk with your health care professional or health care team about when you should eat or drink. The best time to have meals and snacks may depend on

- what medicines you take for diabetes
- what your level of physical activity or your work schedule is
- whether you have other health conditions or diseases

Ask your health care team if you should eat before, during, or after physical activity. Some diabetes medicines, such as sulfonylureas or insulin, may make your blood glucose level drop too low during exercise or if you skip or delay a meal.

## Plan How Much to Eat or Drink

You may worry that having diabetes means giving up foods and drinks you enjoy. The good news is you can still have your favorite foods and drinks, but you might need to have them in smaller portions or enjoy them less often.

For people who have diabetes, carb counting and the plate method are two common ways to plan how much to eat or drink. Talk with your health care professional or health care team to find a method that works for you.

## Carb Counting

Carbohydrate counting External link, or carb counting, means planning and keeping track of the amount of carbs you eat and drink in each meal or snack. Not all people with diabetes need to count carbs. However, if you take insulin, counting carbs can help you know how much insulin to take.

## Plate Method

The plate method External link helps you control portion sizes without counting and measuring. This method divides a 9-inch plate into the following three sections to help you choose the types and amounts of foods External link to eat for each meal.

- Nonstarchy vegetables—such as leafy greens, peppers, carrots, or green beans—should make up half of your plate.
- Carb foods that are high in fiber—such as brown rice, whole grains, beans, or fruits—should make up one-quarter of your plate.
- Protein foods—such as lean meats, fish, dairy, or tofu or other soy products—should make up one quarter of your plate.

If you are not taking insulin, you may not need to count carbs when using the plate method.

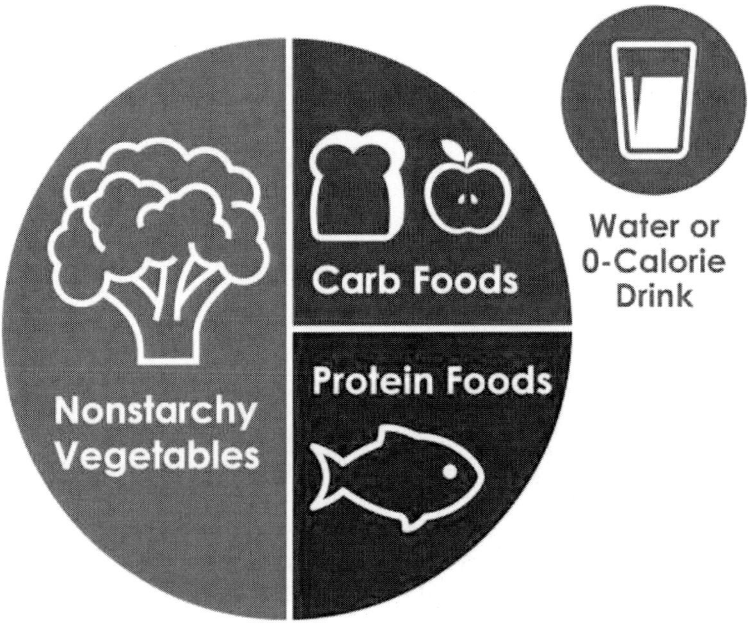


Source: Centers for Disease Control and Prevention The plate method may help you control your blood glucose without counting carbs.

Work with your health care team to create a meal plan that works for you. You may want to have a diabetes educator or a registered dietitian on your team. A registered dietitian can provide medical nutrition therapy External link, which includes counseling to help you create and follow a meal plan. Your health care team may be able to recommend other resources, such as a healthy lifestyle coach, to help you with making changes. Ask your health care team or your insurance company if your benefits include medical nutrition therapy or other diabetes care resources.

## Talk with Your Health Care Professional Before Taking Dietary Supplements

There is no clear proof that specific foods, herbs, spices, or dietary supplements NIH external link—such as vitamins or minerals—can help manage diabetes. Your health care professional may ask you to take vitamins or minerals if you can't get enough from foods. Talk with your health care professional before you take any supplements, because some may cause side effects or affect how well your diabetes medicines work.

## How Can Physical Activity Help Manage My Diabetes?

Research shows that regular physical activity helps people manage their diabetes and stay healthy. Benefits of physical activity may include

- lower blood glucose, blood pressure, and cholesterol levels
- better heart health
- healthier weight
- better mood and sleep
- better balance and memory

Talk with your health care professional before starting a new physical activity or changing how much physical activity you do. They may suggest types of activities based on your ability, schedule, meal plan, interests, and diabetes medicines. Your health care professional may also tell you the best times of day to be active or what to do if your blood glucose level goes out of the range recommended for you.

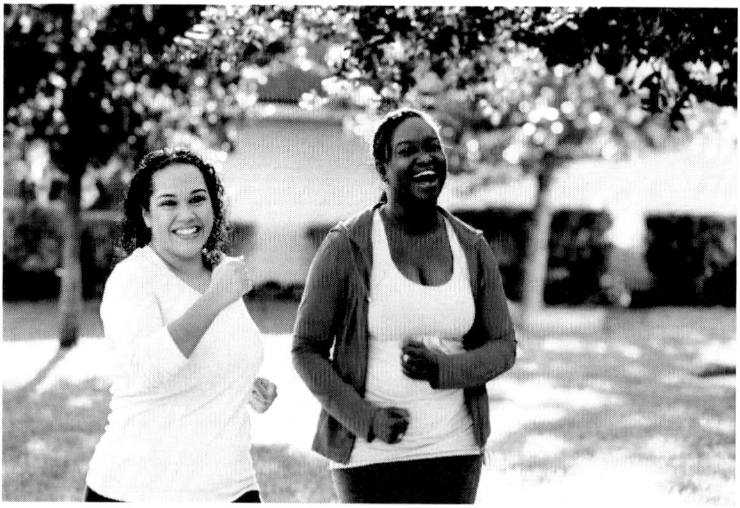

Physical activity may help you manage your diabetes and stay healthy.

## Do Different Types of Physical Activity

People with diabetes can be active, even if they take insulin or use technology such as insulin pumps.

Try to do different kinds of activities. While being more active may have more health benefits, any physical activity is better than none. Start slowly with activities you enjoy. You may be able to change your level of effort and try other activities over time. Having a friend or family member join you may help you stick to your routine.

The physical activities you do may need to be different if you are age 65 or older External link, are pregnant External link, or have a disability or health condition External link. Physical activities may also need to be different for children and teens External link. Ask your health care professional or health care team about activities that are safe for you.

### Aerobic Activities

Aerobic activities make you breathe harder and make your heart beat faster. You can try walking, dancing, wheelchair rolling, or swimming. Most adults should try to get at least 150 minutes of moderate-intensity physical activity External link each week. Aim to do 30 minutes a day on most days of the week. You don't have to do all 30 minutes at one time. You can break up physical activity into small amounts during your day and still get the benefit [1].

### Strength Training or Resistance Training

Strength training or resistance training may make your muscles and bones stronger. You can try lifting weights or doing other exercises such as wall pushups or arm raises. Try to do this kind of training two times a week [1].

### Balance and Stretching Activities

Balance and stretching activities NIH external link may help you move better and have stronger muscles and bones. You may want to try standing on one leg or stretching your legs when sitting on the floor. Try to do these kinds of activities two or three times a week [1].

Some activities that need balance may be unsafe for people with nerve damage or vision problems caused by diabetes. Ask your health care professional or health care team about activities that are safe for you.

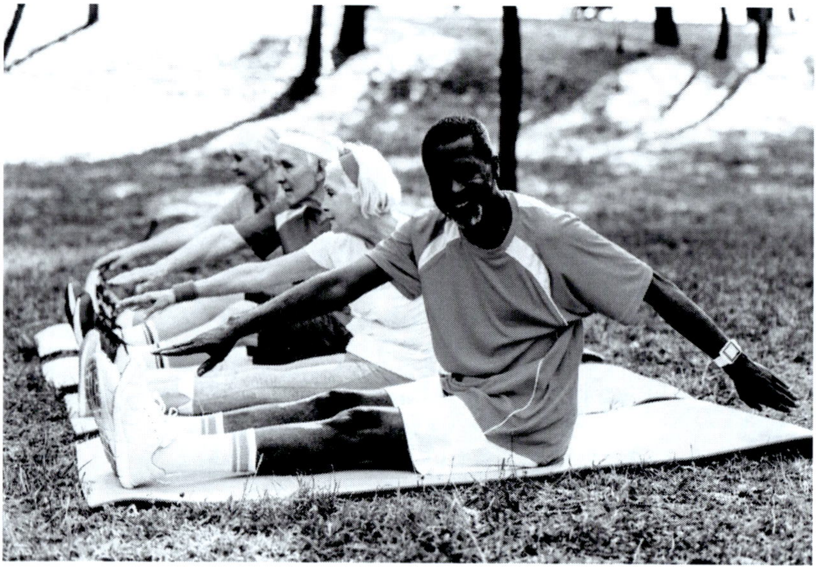

If you can, try to do different types of physical activities. Start slowly with activities you enjoy.

## Stay Safe During Physical Activity

Staying safe during physical activity is important. Here are some tips to keep in mind.

## Drink Liquids

Drinking liquids helps prevent dehydration *NIH external link*, or the loss of too much water in your body. Drinking water is a way to stay hydrated. Sports drinks often have a lot of sugar and calories, and you don't need them for most moderate physical activities.

## Avoid Low Blood Glucose

Check your blood glucose level before, during, and right after physical activity. Physical activity often lowers the level of glucose in your blood. Low blood glucose levels may last for hours or days after physical activity. You are most likely to have low blood glucose if you take insulin or some other diabetes medicines, such as sulfonylureas.

Ask your health care professional if you should take less insulin or eat carbs before, during, or after physical activity. Low blood glucose can be a serious medical emergency that must be treated right away. Take steps to protect yourself. You can learn how to treat low blood glucose, let other people know what to do if you need help, and use a medical alert bracelet.

## Avoid High Blood Glucose and Ketoacidosis

Taking less insulin before physical activity may help prevent low blood glucose, but it may also make you more likely to have high blood glucose. If your body does not have enough insulin, it can't use glucose as a source of energy and will use fat instead. When your body uses fat for energy, your body makes chemicals called ketones.

High levels of ketones in your blood can lead to a condition called diabetic ketoacidosis (DKA) External link. DKA is a medical emergency that should be treated right away. DKA is most common in people with type 1 diabetes. Occasionally, DKA may affect people with type 2 diabetes who have lost their ability to produce insulin. Ask your health care professional how much insulin you should take before physical activity, whether you need to test your urine for ketones, and what level of ketones is dangerous for you.

## Take Care of Your Feet

People with diabetes may have problems with their feet because high blood glucose levels can damage blood vessels and nerves. To help prevent foot problems, wear comfortable and supportive shoes and take care of your feet before, during, and after physical activity.

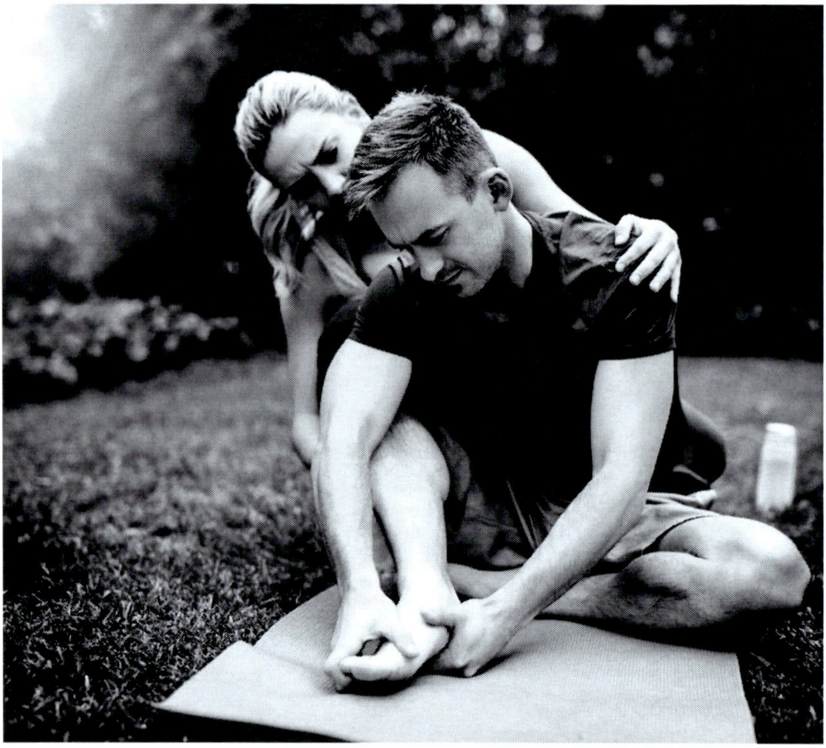

Take care of your feet before, during, and after physical activity.

## What Can I Do to Reach or Maintain a Healthy Weight?

If you have diabetes, managing your weight may bring you several health benefits. Ask your health care professional or health care team if you are at a healthy weight or if you should try to lose weight.

If you are an adult with overweight or obesity, work with your health care team to create a weight-loss plan. Losing 5% to 7% of your current weight may help you prevent or improve some health problems and manage your blood glucose, cholesterol, and blood pressure levels [2]. If you are worried about your child's weight and they have diabetes, talk with their health care professional before your child starts a new weight-loss plan.

You may be able to reach and maintain a healthy weight by

- following a healthy meal plan
- consuming fewer calories
- being physically active
- getting 7 to 8 hours of sleep each night [3]

If you have type 2 diabetes, your health care professional may recommend diabetes medicines that may help you lose weight.

Online tools such as the Body Weight Planner may help you create eating and physical activity plans. You may want to talk with your health care professional about other options for managing your weight, including joining a weight-loss program that can provide helpful information, support, and behavioral or lifestyle counseling. These options may have a cost, so make sure to check the details of the programs.

Your health care professional may recommend weight-loss surgery if you aren't able to reach a healthy weight with meal planning, physical activity, and taking diabetes medicines that help with weight loss.

If you are pregnant, trying to lose weight may not be healthy. However, you should ask your health care professional whether it makes sense to monitor or limit your weight gain during pregnancy.

## Should I Quit Smoking?

Both diabetes and smoking External link—including using tobacco products and e-cigarettes—cause your blood vessels to narrow. Both diabetes and smoking increase your risk of having a heart attack or stroke, nerve damage, kidney disease, eye disease, or amputation. Secondhand smoke External link can also affect the health of your family or others who live with you.

If you smoke or use other tobacco products, stop. Ask for help External link. You don't have to do it alone.

## How Can I Take Care of My Mental Health?

Feeling stressed, sad, or angry can be common for people with diabetes. Managing diabetes or learning to cope with new information about your health can be hard. People with chronic illnesses such as diabetes may develop anxiety or other mental health conditions External link.

Learn healthy ways to lower your stress NIH external link, and ask for help from your health care team or a mental health professional. While it may be uncomfortable to talk about your feelings, finding a health care professional whom you trust and want to talk with may help you

- lower your feelings of stress, depression, or anxiety
- manage problems sleeping or remembering things
- see how diabetes affects your family, school, work, or financial situation

Ask your health care team for mental health resources for people with diabetes.

Sleeping too much or too little External link may raise your blood glucose levels. Your sleep habits may also affect your mental health and vice versa. People with diabetes and overweight or obesity can also have other health conditions that affect sleep, such as sleep apnea NIH external link, which can raise your blood pressure and risk of heart disease.

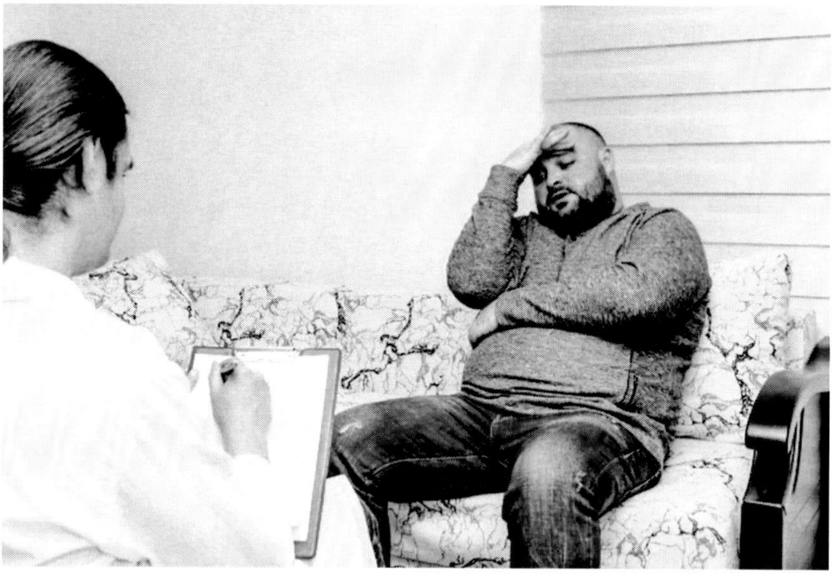

Having diabetes can be stressful. Talk with your health care professional or health care team if you need help.

## Clinical Trials for Healthy Living with Diabetes

NIDDK conducts and supports clinical trials in many diseases and conditions, including diabetes. The trials look to find new ways to prevent, detect, or treat disease and improve quality of life.

## What Are Clinical Trials for Healthy Living with Diabetes?

Clinical trials—and other types of clinical studies NIH external link—are part of medical research and involve people like you. When you volunteer to take part in a clinical study, you help health care professionals and researchers learn more about disease and improve health care for people in the future.

Researchers are studying many aspects of healthy living for people with diabetes, such as

- how changing when you eat may affect body weight and metabolism
- how less access to healthy foods may affect diabetes management, other health problems, and risk of dying
- whether low-carbohydrate meal plans can help lower blood glucose levels
- which diabetes medicines are more likely to help people lose weight

Find out if clinical trials are right for you *NIH external link*.

Watch a video of NIDDK Director Dr. Griffin P. Rodgers explaining the importance of participating in clinical trials.

## What Clinical Trials For Healthy Living with Diabetes Are Looking for Participants?

You can view a filtered list of clinical studies on healthy living with diabetes that are federally funded, open, and recruiting at www.ClinicalTrials.gov *NIH external link*. You can expand or narrow the list to include clinical studies from industry, universities, and individuals; however, the National Institutes of Health does not review these studies and cannot ensure they are safe for you. Always talk with your primary health care professional before you participate in a clinical study.

## References

[1] Office of Disease Prevention and Health Promotion, US Department of Health and Human Services. Physical Activity Guidelines for Americans. 2nd ed. US Department of Health and Human Services; 2018. Accessed March 30, 2023. https://health.gov/paguidelines/ second-edition/ External link.

[2] ElSayed NA, Aleppo G, Aroda VR, et al. Facilitating positive health behaviors and well-being to improve health outcomes: standards of care in diabetes—2023. Diabetes Care. 2023;46(suppl 1):S68–S96. doi:10.2337/dc23-S005.

[3] Watson NF, Badr MS, Belenky G, et al. Recommended amount of sleep for a healthy adult: a joint consensus statement of the American Academy of Sleep Medicine and Sleep Research Society. Sleep. 2015;38(6):843–844. doi:10.5665/sleep.4716.

# Chapter 6

# Managing Diabetes*

## National Institute of Diabetes and Digestive and Kidney Diseases

Diabetes can affect almost every part of your body, including your heart, eyes, kidneys, and nerves. Diabetes is also linked to some types of cancer. You may be able to prevent or delay diabetes health problems by leading a healthy lifestyle, taking your medicines, and managing your blood glucose level, also called blood sugar level. Work with your health care team to create a diabetes care plan that works for you.

## What are the Diabetes ABCs?

The diabetes ABCs can help you manage your blood glucose, blood pressure, and cholesterol levels. If you smoke, quitting is also important. Managing your ABCs may lower your chances of having health problems from diabetes, such as a heart attack, stroke, kidney disease, blindness, and foot or leg amputations.

* This is an edited, reformatted and augmented version of National Institute of Diabetes and Digestive and Kidney Diseases Publication.

In: Comprehensive Diabetes Care
Editor: Joseph S. Green
ISBN: 979-8-89530-772-4

## A is for the A1C Blood Glucose Test

The A1C test shows your average blood glucose level over the last 3 months. This test is done at a health care professional's office or lab. For most people with diabetes, their goal is an A1C level below 7% [1]. Your A1C goal may be different if you have other health problems [2]. Ask your health care team how often you should have the test and what your goal should be.

## B Is for Blood Pressure

High blood pressure NIH external link can damage your heart, kidneys, brain, and eyes. Some people with diabetes have a blood pressure goal below 130/80 mm Hg [2, 3]. If you have heart disease or are at high risk for diabetes health problems, your goal may be lower. Ask your health care team what your goal should be.

## C is for Cholesterol

Cholesterol NIH external link is a fat, also called lipid, that is produced by your liver. Unhealthy levels of cholesterol in your blood can build up and clog your blood vessels, which may result in a heart attack or a stroke. Ask your health care team how often you need a cholesterol test NIH external link, also called a lipid panel, and what your cholesterol level should be. Some people may need to take a medicine called a statin External link, or another medicine, to lower their cholesterol for heart health.

## S is for Stop Smoking

Not smoking is important for your health, especially if you have diabetes. Both smoking and diabetes can make your blood vessels narrow. E-cigarettes aren't a safe option either. If you smoke, vape, or use other tobacco products, stop. Ask for help External link so you don't have to do it alone.

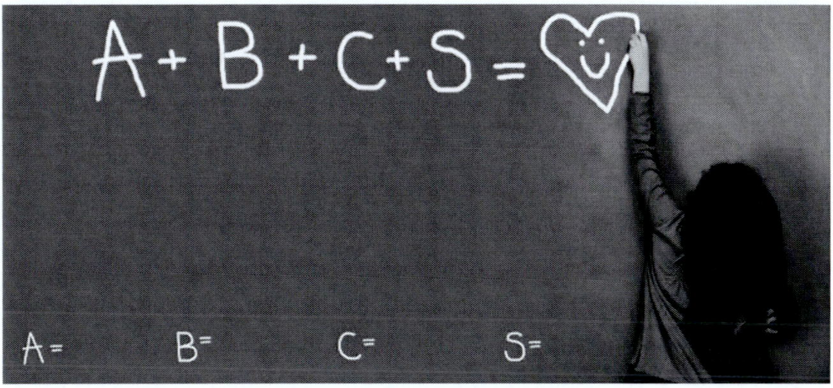


Follow your ABCs to keep your heart healthy. A is for the A1C blood glucose test, B is for blood pressure, C is for cholesterol, and S is for stop smoking.

## How Can a Healthy Lifestyle Help Manage My Diabetes?

Staying healthy when you have diabetes can be a challenge. But leading a healthy lifestyle may help keep your blood glucose, blood pressure, and cholesterol levels in the ranges recommended by your health care team.

## Create a Healthy Meal Plan

You may worry that having diabetes means going without foods you enjoy. The good news is that you can still eat your favorite foods, but you might need to eat smaller portions or enjoy them less often. Work with your health care team, which may include a registered dietitian or a diabetes educator, to create a meal plan that works for you.

Talk with your health care team about any challenges you may have finding healthy food External link. A doctor, registered dietician, diabetes educator, or social worker may be able to recommend resources that can help you. The U.S. Department of Agriculture also provides a list of resources External link about affording healthy food and finding help from food assistance programs.

## Get Physical Activity

Physical activity may help you lower blood glucose, blood pressure, and cholesterol levels. Being active may also help you get better sleep and improve your mood. Try to get at least 150 minutes of moderate-intensity External link physical activity, such as brisk walking, each week. If you can, try to do muscle-strengthening activities, such as wall push-ups or seated arm raises, two days a week [4].

## Reach and Maintain a Healthy Weight

If you are overweight or have obesity, ask your health care team how you can manage your weight. To lose weight, you may need to consume fewer calories or get more physical activity. Your health care team may also recommend medicines or surgery to help manage your weight.

## Get Enough Sleep

Getting enough sleep may improve your mood, energy level, and blood glucose level. Most adults should aim for about 7 to 8 hours each night [5]. Children and adolescents may need more sleep.

## Take Care of Your Mental Health

Feeling stressed, sad, or angry can be common for people with diabetes. Many people with chronic, or long-term, illnesses such as diabetes develop anxiety or other mental health conditions NIH external link. Learn healthy ways to lower your stress NIH external link, and ask for help from your health care team or a mental health professional.

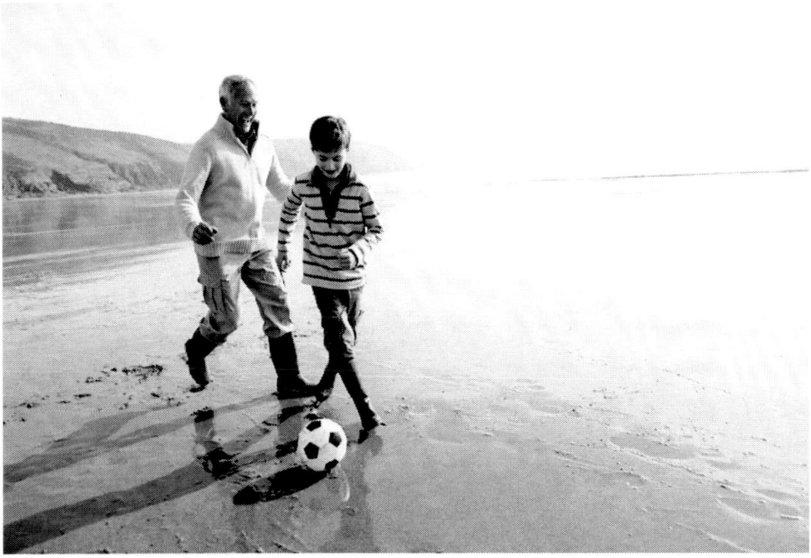

Being physically active can help you manage your diabetes.

## What Types of Medicines Should I Take?

Taking diabetes medicines is often part of managing diabetes. The medicines you take depend on your type of diabetes, how well medicines control your blood glucose level, and other health conditions you may have. You may also need medicines to help manage blood pressure or cholesterol levels. Other factors such as medicine costs, insurance coverage, who is providing your diabetes care, and your lifestyle can also affect what medicines you take.

Take your medicines as they were prescribed, even if you feel good or have reached your blood glucose, blood pressure, or cholesterol goals. Avoid rationing your medicines or skipping taking your medicines if you have trouble paying for them. Talk with your health care team if you can't afford your medicines or if you experience any side effects.

## How Can I Check My Blood Glucose Level at Home?

If you take insulin or other diabetes medicines, checking your blood glucose level at home may help you avoid high or low blood glucose levels. Even if you do not use insulin, checking your blood glucose level at home can help you manage your diabetes. The test results may help you and your health care team make changes to your meal plan, physical activity level, or diabetes medicines. It may help you understand how certain types of food affect your blood glucose level. You do not get the same level of detail from blood tests—such as the A1C test—that you take at a health care professional's office.

If you have type 1 diabetes, your health care team may ask you to check your urine at home for substances called ketones. A large amount of ketones in your urine may mean that you need to manage your diabetes more carefully. Work with your primary health care professional—who may be a doctor, physician assistant, or nurse practitioner—to change your diabetes care plan. If high levels of ketones are left untreated, you may develop a dangerous condition called diabetic ketoacidosis External link.

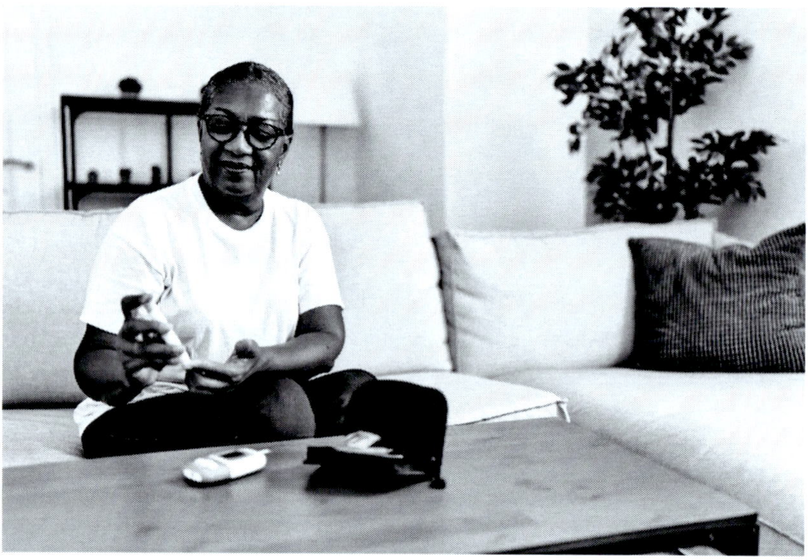

Checking and recording your blood glucose level is an important part of managing diabetes.

## Devices to Help Manage Diabetes

You can check your blood glucose level at home with a blood glucose meter External link. The meter tests a drop of your blood, usually from a prick of your fingertip. The meter will show you how much glucose is in your blood at that moment.

People who take insulin to manage their diabetes may benefit from using a continuous glucose monitor (CGM). A CGM uses a sensor in the tissue under your skin and shows changes in glucose levels throughout the day and night. Many CGM systems have alarms and warnings that let you know if your glucose level is too low or too high.

For safety, you may sometimes need to compare your CGM glucose readings with results from a standard blood glucose meter. This could be needed if you doubt the accuracy of your CGM readings, if you are changing your insulin dose, or if your CGM gives a warning alert.

Some people use a CGM as part of an artificial pancreas. An artificial pancreas is a system that mimics how a healthy pancreas controls blood glucose in the body. A CGM, an insulin pump, and a software program that shares information between the CGM and insulin pump make up the artificial pancreas.

Ask your health care team about the best way to check your blood glucose level and how often you should check it. Make sure to keep a record of your blood glucose self-checks, including the date and time you checked it, the results, and other information, such as what you ate or what physical activity you did that day. You can use a chart or a smartphone app to help you keep track. Take this information with you when you visit your health care team.

## Recommended Targets for Blood Glucose Levels

Talk with your health care team about the blood glucose range that is healthy for you. Be sure to tell your health care team if your glucose levels frequently go above or below your target range.

Many people with diabetes aim to keep their blood glucose at these levels [1].

- Before a meal: 80 to 130 mg/dL
- About 2 hours after a meal starts: less than 180 mg/dL

Your blood glucose goals may be different if you are an adult over age 65 and have had diabetes for a long time. Your blood glucose goals may also be different if you have other health problems, like heart disease, or if your blood glucose often gets too low.

If you use a CGM, your health care team may ask you to keep track of your time in range. Time in range is the percentage of time that your glucose level stays in your target range. For many people with diabetes, the target range is between 70 and 180 mg/dL. Your health care team may adjust your diabetes care plan to help you stay in your target range at least 70% of the time.

## Low Blood Glucose

When your blood glucose level is too low, it is called hypoglycemia. For most people with diabetes, the blood glucose level is too low when it is below 70 mg/dL.[1,2] Talk with your primary care professional or health care team if you often have low blood glucose levels. Some people with low blood glucose experience symptoms such as

- feeling shaky or jittery
- headache
- cold sweat

If you often have low blood glucose levels, you may need to change your diabetes meal plan, physical activity plan, or medicines. Very low blood glucose may lead to confusion or fainting NIH external link, and it can become a serious medical emergency that must be treated right away.

Glucagon—a hormone that raises blood glucose levels—is the best way to treat severely low blood glucose. Ask your health care team if you need a prescription for glucagon. If you have a glucagon prescription, you should teach your family, friends, and coworkers when and how to give you glucagon in case you are not able to do it yourself.

## High Blood Glucose

When your blood glucose level is too high, it is called hyperglycemia. For most people with diabetes, the blood glucose level is too high when it is above

180 mg/dL. Talk with your health care team if you often have high blood glucose levels. Some people with high blood glucose have symptoms such as

- feeling tired
- feeling thirsty
- having blurry vision
- urinating too often

If you often have high blood glucose levels, you may need to make a change to your diabetes meal plan, physical activity plan, or medicines. Very high blood glucose may lead to confusion or fainting, and it may become a serious medical emergency that must be treated right away.

## Checking Urine for Ketones

Your health care team may want you to check your urine for ketones if you have symptoms of diabetic ketoacidosis. Diabetic ketoacidosis is a medical emergency that needs to be treated right away.

Symptoms of diabetic ketoacidosis include

- feeling very tired
- having trouble breathing
- having fruity-smelling breath
- fainting

Most often, ketoacidosis affects people with type 1 diabetes. However, some people with type 2 diabetes can develop ketoacidosis if they do not produce enough insulin.

## How Can I Keep Track of My Progress?

You may find it helpful to keep track of your ABCs and other important health information that you get during checkups with your primary care professional or other health care professionals. Download the Health Checkups Tracker (DOCX, 67.97 KB) , which includes information you may want to track. You can take this information with you when you visit your health care team. Talk with your primary care professional about your goals and whether you need to make any changes to your diabetes care plan.

## What Special Situations Should I Plan for?

If you have diabetes, it is important to take care of your health no matter what is going on in your life. Ask your health care team if you should adjust your meal plan, activity level, or medicines in special situations, such as when you are sick External link, fasting, at school External link, planning to travel External link, or experiencing an emergency or natural disaster External link.

## Who Should Be on My Health Care Team?

You are the most important member of your health care team, but working with your health care team may help you improve your self-care. Most people with diabetes get help from a primary care professional, such as an internal medicine doctor, family doctor, pediatrician, physician assistant, or certified nurse practitioner trained in diabetes care. Ask your primary care professional about adding other members to your team, including

- a diabetes educator, nurse, or registered dietitian who can tell you more about your disease External link and how to improve your self-care
- a dentist to check for gum diseases and other dental problems
- an eye doctor to check for diabetic eye disease
- a pharmacist to help you with your medicines
- other specialists if you develop health problems such as heart disease, kidney disease, erectile dysfunction, or foot problems
- a social worker who may be able to help you find financial help for diabetes care and community resources

Write a list of questions External link before your visit with a health care professional so you don't forget what you want to ask.

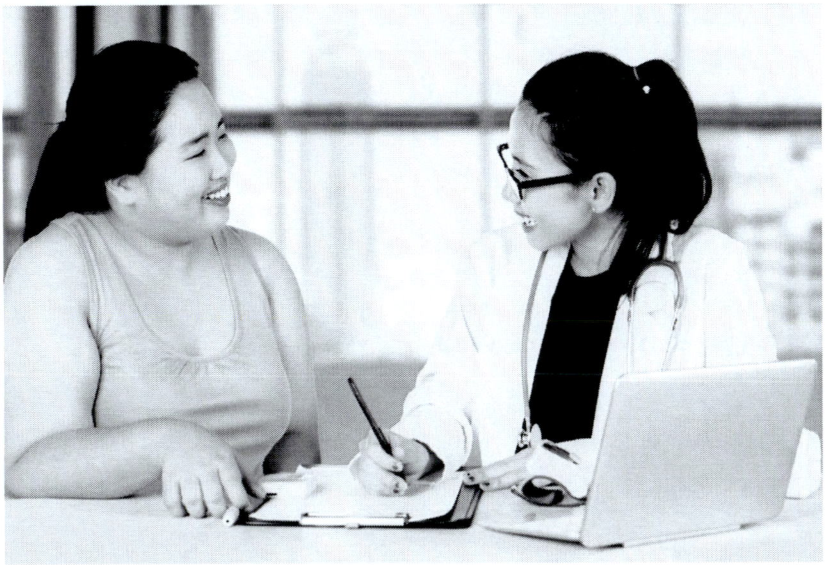

When you see your health care professional, discuss your diabetes self-care plan, review your blood glucose chart or app, and ask questions.

## Clinical Trials for Managing Diabetes

NIDDK conducts and supports clinical trials in many diseases and conditions, including diabetes. The trials look to find new ways to prevent, detect, or treat diseases and improve quality of life.

## What Are Clinical Trials for Managing Diabetes?

Clinical trials—and other types of clinical studies *NIH external link*—are part of medical research and involve people like you. When you volunteer to take part in a clinical study, you help health care professionals and researchers learn more about diseases and improve health care for people in the future.

Researchers are studying many aspects of managing diabetes, such as

- what are the best medicines to add to a diabetes care plan if a person with type 2 diabetes isn't meeting their blood glucose targets using their current diabetes medicines
- how to train adolescents to support or care for family members with diabetes
- how treating obesity with weight-loss medicines or weight-loss surgery, also called metabolic and bariatric surgery, may help manage type 2 diabetes
- what different devices can help people with diabetes check their blood glucose level and inject insulin

Find out if clinical trials are right for you NIH external link.

Watch a video of NIDDK Director Dr. Griffin P. Rodgers explaining the importance of participating in clinical trials.

## What Clinical Trials for Managing Diabetes Are Looking for Participants?

You can view a filtered list of clinical studies on managing diabetes that are federally funded, open, and recruiting at www.ClinicalTrials.gov *NIH external link*. You can expand or narrow the list to include clinical studies from industry, universities, and individuals; however, the National Institutes of Health does not review these studies and cannot ensure they are safe for you. Always talk with your primary health care professional before you participate in a clinical study.

## What Have We Learned About Managing Diabetes from NIDDK-Funded Research?

The research funded by NIDDK has improved quality of life for people with diabetes by finding better ways to diagnose and treat the disease.

## Artificial Pancreas

For decades, NIDDK has supported research that helped create artificial pancreas technology used by some people who need insulin to manage their diabetes.

NIDDK supported research that helped scientists develop the first continuous glucose monitor (CGM) that was approved by the U.S. Food and Drug Administration (FDA) in 1999. CGMs, which are part of artificial pancreas systems, help people track glucose levels in real-time with fewer finger pricks. Another major milestone came in 2016, when the FDA approved a commercial "hybrid" artificial pancreas system. Other artificial pancreas systems have been approved since 2016. NIDDK continues to support research into artificial pancreas systems and other technologies that may improve diabetes management.

## Blood Glucose Management Studies

NIDDK funded the landmark Diabetes Control and Complications Trial (DCCT). The study showed that participants with type 1 diabetes who kept their blood glucose levels close to normal greatly lowered their chances of developing eye, kidney, and nerve disease. A follow-up study, the ongoing Epidemiology of Diabetes Interventions and Complications (EDIC) study External link, has continued to follow DCCT participants since 1994. EDIC has shown that there are long-term benefits of early and intensive blood glucose management on slowing or preventing the development of health problems such as heart, eye, kidney, and nerve diseases. Findings from the DCCT and EDIC studies changed the way diabetes is treated worldwide, and they show that blood glucose control can help people with diabetes lead longer and healthier lives.

NIDDK also funded the Diabetes & Aging Study to research the effects of early blood glucose management and the development of diabetes health problems in people with type 2 diabetes. The study found that people with less effective diabetes management during the first year after being diagnosed with diabetes had a higher risk of diabetes complications and death.

The Treatment Options for Type 2 Diabetes in Adolescents and Youth (TODAY) study and a follow-up study, TODAY2, found that type 2 diabetes can be more difficult to treat and manage when it occurs in younger people.

The TODAY studies, both funded by NIDDK, show the importance of early, intensive treatment and blood glucose management for children or adolescents diagnosed with type 2 diabetes.

## References

[1] ElSayed NA, Aleppo G, Aroda VR, et al. 6. Glycemic targets: standards of care in diabetes—2023. *Diabetes Care*. 2023;46(suppl 1):S97–S110. doi:10.2337/dc23-S006.

[2] Blonde L, Umpierrez GE, Reddy SS, et al. American Association of Clinical Endocrinology clinical practice guideline: developing a diabetes mellitus comprehensive care plan—2022 update. *Endocrine Practice*. 2022; 28(10):923–1049. doi:10.1016/j.eprac.2022.08.002.

[3] ElSayed NA, Aleppo G, Aroda VR, et al. 10. Cardiovascular disease and risk management: standards of care in diabetes—2023. *Diabetes Care*. 2023;46(suppl 1):S158–S190. doi:10.2337/dc23-S010.

[4] Office of Disease Prevention and Health Promotion, US Department of Health and Human Services. *Physical Activity Guidelines for Americans*. 2nd ed. US Department of Health and Human Services; 2018. Accessed March 30, 2023. https://health.gov/paguidelines/second-edition/ External link.

[5] Watson NF, Badr MS, Belenky G, et al. Recommended amount of sleep for a healthy adult: a joint consensus statement of the American Academy of Sleep Medicine and Sleep Research Society. *Sleep*. 2015;38(6):843–844. doi:10.5665/sleep.4716.

Chapter 7

# Managing Diabetes: New Technologies Can Make It Easier*

National Institutes of Health

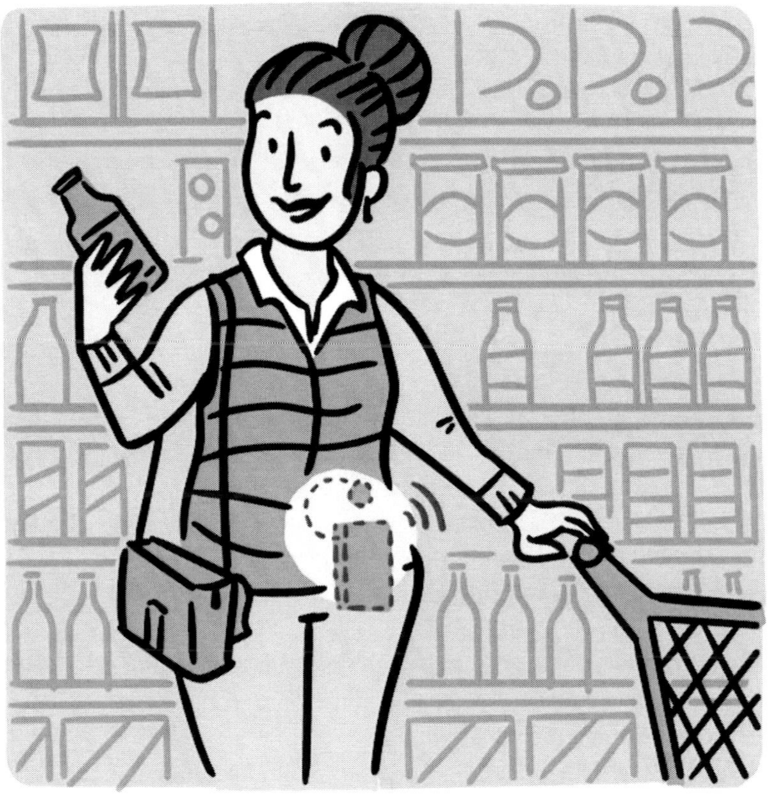

* This is an edited, reformatted and augmented version of National Institutes of Health Plication.

In: Comprehensive Diabetes Care
Editor: Joseph S. Green
ISBN: 979-8-89530-772-4

Your body takes care of countless tasks for you. You might not notice all it's doing to keep you healthy until something goes wrong.

Diabetes is a serious disease that happens when your body has trouble managing and using blood glucose, a sugar that your body uses as fuel. When you have diabetes, you must actively take on this process yourself. New technologies are being tested to make it easier for you to control diabetes and to help you stay healthy.

More than 100 million Americans are living with diabetes or prediabetes, a condition where blood glucose levels are higher than normal, but not high enough to be considered diabetes. People with diabetes must frequently check their blood glucose (or blood sugar) and take quick action if it gets too high or low. They must also constantly consider how all meals, physical activity, and things like stress will affect their blood glucose.

## Types of Diabetes

How people with diabetes manage their blood glucose levels depends, in part, on the type of diabetes they have. The most common are type 1, type 2, and gestational diabetes.

With type 1 diabetes, your body doesn't make enough of a hormone called insulin. Insulin signals the body's cells to let glucose inside. The body can't produce enough insulin because the immune system, your body's defense against germs and foreign substances, mistakenly attacks and destroys the cells in your pancreas that make insulin.

Type 2 diabetes is the most common. It occurs when either your body's cells have trouble using insulin or your body doesn't produce enough insulin to handle the glucose in your blood.

Both types can develop at any age. Type 1 is most often diagnosed in children and young adults, while type 2 shows up most in middle-age and older people. Gestational diabetes occurs only during pregnancy, but increases your chances of developing type 2 later in life.

Diabetes symptoms can vary by type. Some shared symptoms include increased thirst, hunger, and urination. Symptoms of type 1 can start quickly, over a few weeks. Type 2 symptoms tend to develop slowly over years, making them less noticeable.

## Blood Glucose Control

Many people with diabetes check their blood glucose with a blood glucose meter. This portable machine measures how much glucose is in the blood. You get a drop of blood by pricking the side of your fingertip with a small, specialized needle. Then you apply the blood to a test strip. The meter shows you how much glucose is in your blood at that moment.

People with type 1 diabetes, and some people with type 2, correct and manage their blood glucose with injections of synthetic insulin. A missed, or miscalculated, dose can lead to serious complications, immediately and over time. Diabetes increases your risk for blindness, heart disease, stroke, kidney failure, and amputation.

"It's a significant burden to self-test sugar levels several times a day, count carbohydrates with each meal, take into account the impact of physical activity, and then calculate the amount of insulin you need to inject multiple times a day with a syringe or the help of an insulin pump," explains Dr. Guillermo Arreaza-Rubín, who heads NIH's Diabetes Technology Program. Any error in this management may lead to life-threatening complications like severe hypoglycemia, which is very low blood glucose.

"Hypoglycemia is one of the main reasons people with type 1 visit hospital emergency rooms every day," Arreaza-Rubín says. "It happens more frequently during the night and is a major cause of fear and anxiety among people with diabetes and their families."

## Help From Technology

NIH funded-scientists are testing promising technologies to help people better manage diabetes. For example, "artificial pancreas" systems monitor blood glucose levels and provide insulin, or a combination of insulin and another important hormone, automatically. The devices vary in how easy they are to set up and use.

"Our device, called the iLet, is designed to minimize the guesswork and time drain that comes with managing type 1 diabetes," says Dr. Edward Damiano, a biomedical engineering expert at Boston University who's co-founded a company to further develop the technology. The device only requires that you type in your body weight to get started. "The system does the heavy lifting of regulating blood glucose, freeing up the user to live a less burdened and more spontaneous life."

Previous studies have shown that artificial pancreas systems can be safer than the current standard for insulin delivery. Several different devices are now being tested in more people for longer periods of time. Researchers are looking at safety, user-friendliness, the physical and emotional health of the participants, and cost.

Safety is a priority for researchers. "When people with type 1 exercise, their blood glucose can respond in unpredictable and potentially dangerous ways," explains University of Virginia engineer Dr. Marc Breton. He led a recent study that showed an artificial pancreas system improved glycemic control and reduced hypoglycemia in adolescents with type 1 diabetes as they participated in winter sports, like skiing and snowboarding.

"The artificial pancreas performed very well in an extremely challenging environment," he says. "Eventually, it may allow people with diabetes the freedom to participate safely in physical activities that they likely avoided in the past."

One FDA-approved artificial pancreas is already available for people with diabetes. Devices that are more fully automated may become available to the public within the next couple years. Researchers are considering how to use these systems for people with type 2, gestational diabetes, and other conditions involving elevated blood glucose levels.

Other scientists are taking different approaches to replace insulin more effectively. For example, "smart insulins" would become active only when needed. Researchers are also looking for ways to regenerate or replace insulin-producing cells—and to stop the body from attacking them.

"These technologies will help make managing diabetes easier and will help make people who use them healthier," says Damiano. "I see them as a bridge to a cure for type 1 diabetes."

While future tools may make it easier to manage your diabetes, you can learn how to manage diabetes with the tools we have now to live a long, healthy life. Medications, glucose monitors, and insulin pumps are all available now to help people with diabetes. If you have diabetes, talk with your health care provider about your options.

# Chapter 8

# Diabetes, Heart Disease, and Stroke*


## National Institute of Diabetes and Digestive and Kidney Diseases


Having diabetes means you are more likely to develop heart disease. People with diabetes are also more likely to have certain risk factors, such as high blood pressure NIH external link or high cholesterol, that increase their chances of having a heart attack or a stroke.

If you have diabetes, you can protect your heart and health by managing your blood glucose, also called blood sugar. You can also protect yourself by controlling your high blood pressure and high cholesterol. If you smoke, get help to stop.

## What Is the Link Between Diabetes, Heart Disease, and Stroke?

High blood glucose from diabetes can damage your blood vessels and the nerves that control your heart and blood vessels. Over time, this damage can lead to heart disease [1].

People with diabetes tend to develop heart disease at a younger age than people without diabetes. Adults with diabetes are nearly twice as likely to have heart disease or stroke as adults without diabetes [2, 3].

---

* This is an edited, reformatted and augmented version of National Institute of Diabetes and Digestive and Kidney Diseases Publication.


In: Comprehensive Diabetes Care
Editor: Joseph S. Green
ISBN: 979-8-89530-772-4

The good news is that the steps you take to manage your diabetes also help lower your chances of having heart disease or stroke.

## What Else Increases My Chances of Heart Disease or Stroke If I Have Diabetes?

Your risk for heart disease is greater if you are male rather than female, whether you have diabetes or not [2]. If you do have diabetes, other factors add to your chances of developing heart disease or having a stroke.

### Smoking

Smoking raises your risk of developing heart disease. If you have diabetes, it is important to stop smoking, because both smoking and diabetes narrow blood vessels. Smoking also increases your chances of developing other long-term problems such as

- lung disease NIH external link
- lower leg infections and ulcers
- foot or leg amputation

### High Blood Pressure

If you have high blood pressure NIH external link, your heart works harder to pump blood. High blood pressure can strain your heart, damage blood vessels, and increase your risk of heart attack, stroke, and eye or kidney problems. Have your blood pressure checked regularly and work with your doctor to control or lower high blood pressure.

### Abnormal Cholesterol Levels

Cholesterol NIH external link is a type of fat, produced by your liver and found in your blood. You have two kinds of cholesterol in your blood: LDL and HDL.

LDL, often called “bad” cholesterol, can build up and clog your blood vessels. High levels of LDL cholesterol raise your risk of developing heart disease. HDL is sometimes called “good cholesterol.” Higher levels of HDL is linked to lower risk for heart disease and stroke. To improve LDL and HDL levels, limit the amount of fat in your eating plan, eat more plant-based foods, and get regular physical activity.

Another type of blood fat, triglycerides, also can raise your risk of heart disease when the levels are higher than recommended by your health care team.

## Obesity and Belly Fat

Being overweight or having obesity can make it harder to manage your diabetes and raise your risk for many health problems, including heart disease and high blood pressure. If you are overweight, a healthy eating plan with fewer calories and more physical activity often will lower your blood glucose levels and reduce your need for medicines.

Excess belly fat around your waist, even if you are not overweight, can raise your chances of developing heart disease.

You have excess belly fat if your waist measures

- more than 40 inches and you are a man
- more than 35 inches and you are a woman

## Chronic Kidney Disease

Heart disease is closely linked with chronic kidney disease, a condition in which your kidneys are damaged and can’t filter blood the way they should. Having diabetes is a risk factor for developing kidney disease, which affects about 40% of people with diabetes. Other risk factors for developing kidney disease are high blood pressure and a family history of kidney failure.

If you have risk factors, get tested for kidney disease and protect your kidneys by making healthy food choices, being more active, aiming for a healthy weight, and managing health conditions that cause kidney damage.

## Family History of Heart Disease

A family history of heart disease may add to your chances of developing the condition. If one or more of your family members had a heart attack before age 50, you have double the chance of developing heart disease compared with people who have no family history of the disease [4].

You can't change whether heart disease runs in your family. But if you have diabetes, it's even more important to take steps to protect yourself from heart disease and decrease your chances of having a stroke.

## How Can I Lower My Chances of a Heart Attack or Stroke If I Have Diabetes?

Taking care of your diabetes is important to help you protect your heart. You can substantially lower your chances of having a heart attack or stroke by taking the following steps to keep your heart and blood vessels healthy [5].

## Manage Your Diabetes ABCs

Know your diabetes ABCs to help you manage your blood glucose, blood pressure, and cholesterol. Stop smoking if you have diabetes to lower your chances of developing heart disease.

## A Is for The A1C Test

The A1C test shows your average blood glucose level over the past 3 months. This is different from the blood glucose checks you do every day. The higher your A1C number, the higher your blood glucose levels have been during the past 3 months. High levels of blood glucose can harm your heart, blood vessels, kidneys, feet, and eyes.

The A1C goal for many people with diabetes is below 7%. Some people may do better with a slightly higher A1C goal. Your A1C goals may also change as you get older and your lifestyle changes. Ask your health care team what your goal should be.

## B Is for Blood Pressure

Blood pressure is the force of your blood against the wall of your blood vessels. If your blood pressure gets too high, it makes your heart work too hard. High blood pressure can cause a heart attack or stroke and damage your kidneys and eyes.

The blood pressure goal for most people with diabetes is below 140/90 mm Hg. Ask what your goal should be.

## C is for Cholesterol

A buildup of cholesterol, a form of fat found in your blood, can cause a heart attack or stroke. Ask your health care team what your cholesterol numbers should be. If you are over 40 years old, you may need to take medicine, such as a statin *NIH external link*, to lower your cholesterol levels and protect your heart. Some people with very high LDL ("bad") cholesterol may need to take medicine starting at a younger age.

Learn about getting your cholesterol checked External link.

## S Is for Stop Smoking

Quitting smoking is especially important for people with diabetes because both smoking and diabetes narrow blood vessels, so your heart has to work harder. E-cigarettes aren't a safe option either.

If you quit smoking

- you will lower your risk for heart attack; stroke; nerve, kidney, and eye disease; and amputation
- your blood glucose, blood pressure, and cholesterol levels may improve
- your blood circulation will improve
- you may have an easier time being physically active

If you smoke or use other tobacco products, stop. Ask for help so you don't have to do it alone. You can start by calling the National Quitline at 1-

800-QUITNOW or 1-800-784-8669. For tips on quitting, go to Smokefree.gov External link.

Ask your health care team about your goals for A1C, blood pressure, and cholesterol, and what you can do to reach these goals. To improve your diabetes self-management skills, you may want a referral to a diabetes educator or a registered dietitian. Medicare, some private insurers, and other organizations will provide financial assistance for some of these services.

You can keep track of your ABCs with a diabetes record form. You can use it when you meet with your health care team in person or remotely. Talk with your team about your goals and how you are doing, and whether you need to make any changes to your diabetes care plan.

## Develop or Maintain Healthy Lifestyle Habits

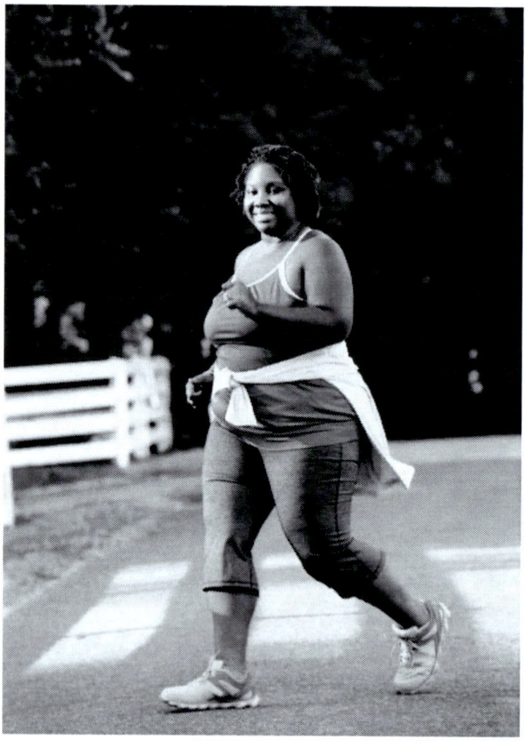

Develop or maintain healthy lifestyle habits. Physical activity can help you manage your diabetes and may help you cope with stress.

Healthy lifestyle habits that you stick with can help you manage your diabetes and prevent heart disease.

- Follow your healthy eating plan.
- Make physical activity part of your routine.
- Stay at or get to a healthy weight.
- Get enough sleep.

Learn more about these tips to manage diabetes.

Watch a video about what you can do to keep your heart healthy External link.

Learn about the Body Weight Planner, which may help you create a personal plan to reach your goal weight.

## Learn to Manage Stress

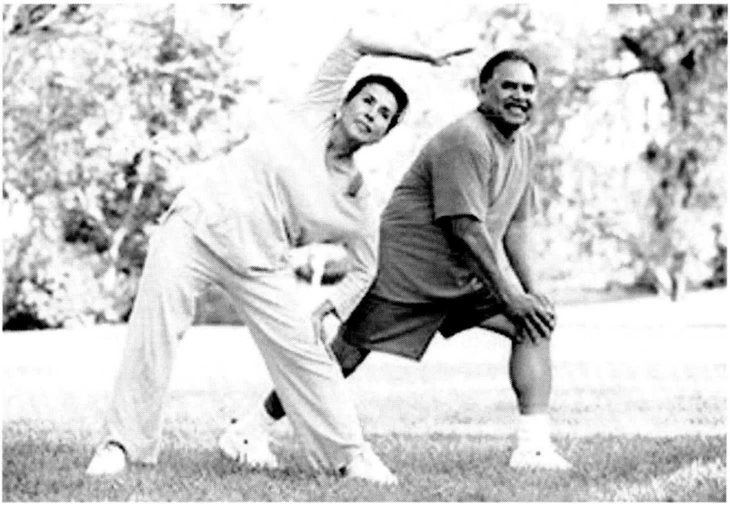

Yoga and other forms of exercise can help reduce stress.

Managing diabetes is not always easy. Feeling stressed, sad, lonely, or angry is common when you are living with diabetes. You may know what to do to stay healthy but may have trouble sticking with your plan over time. Long-term stress can raise your blood glucose and blood pressure, but you can learn ways to lower your stress. Try deep breathing, gardening, taking a walk, doing yoga, talking with a loved one, working on a hobby, or listening to your favorite music. Learn more about healthy ways to cope with stress NIH external link.

## Take Medicine to Protect Your Heart

Medicines may be an important part of your treatment plan. Your doctor will prescribe medicine based on your specific needs. Medicine may help you

- meet your A1C (blood glucose), blood pressure, and cholesterol goals.
- reduce your risk of blood clots, heart attack, or stroke.
- treat angina NIH external link, or chest pain that is often a symptom of heart disease. Angina can also be an early symptom of a heart attack.
- treat heart failure, which is a form of heart disease in which your heart cannot pump blood well enough for your body to work properly.

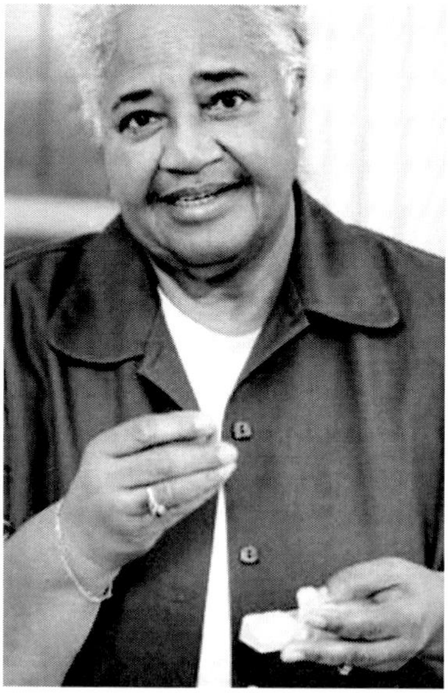

Take medicines as prescribed.

Ask your doctor whether you should take daily aspirin. Aspirin is not safe for everyone. Your doctor can tell you whether taking aspirin is right for you and exactly how much to take.

Statins can reduce the risk of having a heart attack or stroke in some people with diabetes. In addition, certain diabetes medicines have been shown to reduce the risk of heart attacks and death in patients at very high risk of having a heart attack. Talk with your doctor to find out whether taking a statin or a diabetes medicine that reduces heart attack risk is right for you.

Take medicines the way your doctor or health care team tells you to. Talk with your doctor or pharmacist if you have questions about your medicines. Before you start a new medicine, ask your doctor about possible side effects and how you can avoid them. If the side effects of your medicine bother you, tell your doctor. Don't stop taking your medicines without checking with your doctor first.

## How Do Doctors Diagnose Heart Disease in People with Diabetes?

Doctors diagnose heart disease in people with diabetes *NIH external link* based on their

- symptoms
- medical and family history
- how likely they are to have heart disease
- a physical exam
- results from tests and procedures

Tests used to monitor your diabetes—A1C, blood pressure, and cholesterol—help your doctor decide whether it is important to do additional tests to check your heart health or to refer you to a specialist such as a cardiologist.

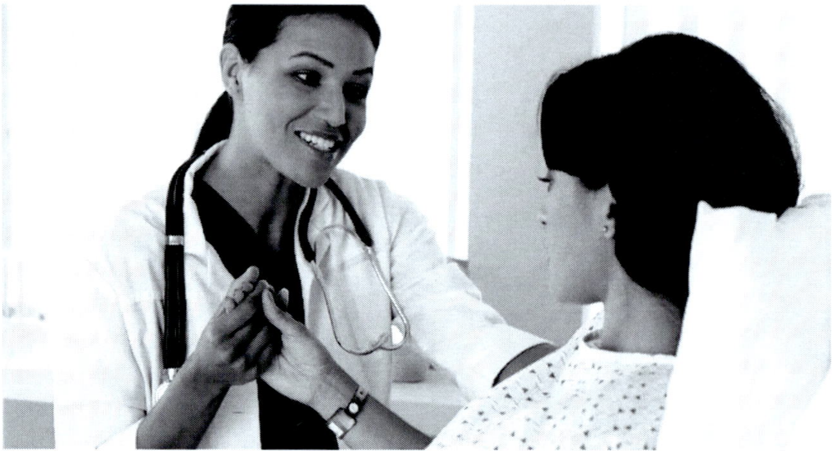

Your health care professional will do a physical exam.
Ask your health care team these questions.

- What can we do to lower my chances of getting heart disease?
- How can we work together to help me maintain my goals for A1C, blood pressure, and cholesterol?
- What medicines, such as aspirin or a statin, will help protect my heart?
- Are there diabetes medicines that will help protect my heart?

## What Are the Warning Signs of Heart Attack and Stroke?

Call 9-1-1 right away if you have any of these warning signs of a heart attack

- pain or pressure in your chest that lasts longer than a few minutes or goes away and comes back
- pain or discomfort in one or both of your arms or shoulders, or your back, neck, or jaw
- shortness of breath
- sweating or light-headedness
- indigestion or nausea (feeling sick to your stomach)
- feeling very tired

Treatment works best when it is given right away. Warning signs can be different in different people. You may not have all the listed symptoms.

Women may experience chest pain, nausea, and vomiting; feel very tired (sometimes for days); and have pain that spreads to the back, neck, throat, arms, shoulders, or jaw. People with diabetes-related nerve damage may not notice any chest pain.

If you have angina *NIH external link*, it's important to know how and when to seek medical treatment.

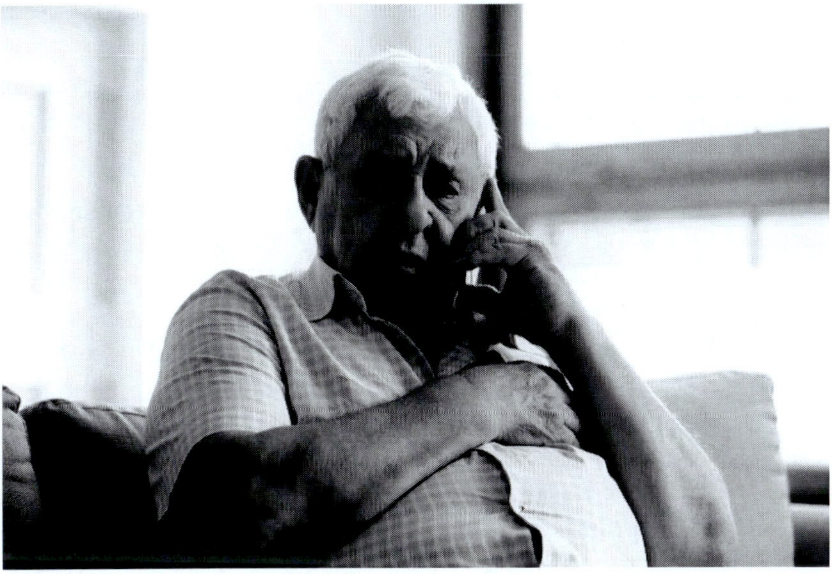

Call 9-1-1 if you have the warning signs of a heart attack or stroke. Treatment works best when given right away.

Call 9-1-1 right away if you have any of these warning signs of a stroke, including sudden

- weakness or numbness of your face, arm, or leg on one side of your body
- confusion, or trouble talking or understanding
- dizziness, loss of balance, or trouble walking
- trouble seeing out of one or both eyes
- sudden, severe headache

If you have any one of these warning signs, call 9-1-1. You can help prevent permanent damage by getting to a hospital within an hour of a stroke.

## Clinical Trials for Diabetes, Heart Disease, & Stroke

The NIDDK conducts and supports clinical trials in many diseases and conditions, including diabetes. The trials look to find new ways to prevent, detect, or treat disease and improve quality of life.

## What Are Clinical Trials for Diabetes, Heart Disease, and Stroke?

Clinical trials—and other types of clinical studies—are part of medical research and involve people like you. When you volunteer to take part in a clinical study, you help doctors and researchers learn more about disease and improve health care for people in the future.

Researchers are studying many aspects of diabetes, heart disease, and stroke, such as

- risk factors for heart disease and stroke in specific populations, such as Black Americans with diabetes
- improved imaging techniques and tests to help diagnose and treat conditions that lead to heart attacks and stroke
- the role of genetics in diabetes, heart disease, and stroke

Find out if clinical studies are right for you NIH external link.

Watch a video of NIDDK Director Dr. Griffin P. Rodgers explaining the importance of participating in clinical trials.

## What Clinical Trials for Heart Disease and Stroke Are Looking for Participants?

You can view a filtered list of clinical studies on diabetes and heart disease that are federally funded, open, and recruiting at www.ClinicalTrials.gov NIH external link. A separate list of clinical studies on diabetes and stroke is also available at www.ClinicalTrials.gov NIH external link. You can expand or narrow the list to include clinical studies from industry, universities, and individuals; however, the National Institutes of Health does not review these studies and cannot ensure they are safe. Always talk with your health care provider before you participate in a clinical study.

## References

[1] Nanayakkara N, Curtis AJ, Heritier S, et al. Impact of age at type 2 diabetes mellitus diagnosis on mortality and vascular complications: systematic review and meta-analyses. *Diabetologia.* 2021;64(2):275–287. doi:10.1007/s00125-020-05319-w.

[2] Barrett-Connor E, Wingard D, Wong N, Goldberg R. Chapter 18: Heart disease and diabetes (PDF, 1.07 MB) . In: Cowie CC, Casagrande SS, Menke A, et al, eds. Diabetes in America, 3rd ed. NIH Pub No. 17-1468. *National Institutes of Health*; 2018:18.1–18.30.

[3] Pikula A, Howard BV, Seshadri S. Chapter 19: Stroke and diabetes (PDF, 493.93 KB) . In: Cowie CC, Casagrande SS, Menke A, et al, eds. Diabetes in America, 3rd ed. NIH Pub No. 17-1468. *National Institutes of Health;* 2018:19.1–19.23.

[4] Moonesinghe R, Yang Q, Zhang Z, Khoury MJ. Prevalence and cardiovascular health impact of family history of premature heart disease in the United States: analysis of the National Health and Nutrition Examination Survey, 2007–2014. *Journal of the American Heart Association.* 2019;8(14):e012364. doi:10.1161/JAHA.119.012364.

[5] Wong ND, Zhao Y, Patel R, et al. Cardiovascular risk factor targets and cardiovascular disease event risk in diabetes: a pooling project of the Atherosclerosis Risk in Communities Study, Multi-Ethnic Study of Atherosclerosis, and Jackson Heart Study. *Diabetes Care*. 2016;39(5):668–676. doi:10.2337/dc15-2439.

# Chapter 9

# Diabetic Kidney Disease*

National Institute of Diabetes and Digestive and Kidney Diseases

## What Is Diabetic Kidney Disease?

Diabetic kidney disease is a type of kidney disease caused by diabetes.

Diabetes is the leading cause of kidney disease. About 1 out of 3 adults with diabetes has kidney disease [1].

The main job of the kidneys is to filter wastes and extra water out of your blood to make urine. Your kidneys also help control blood pressure and make hormones that your body needs to stay healthy.

When your kidneys are damaged, they can't filter blood like they should, which can cause wastes to build up in your body. Kidney damage can also cause other health problems.

Kidney damage caused by diabetes usually occurs slowly, over many years. You can take steps to protect your kidneys and to prevent or delay kidney damage.

Watch a video about diabetes and kidney disease External link.

---

* This is an edited, reformatted and augmented version of National Institute of Diabetes and Digestive and Kidney Diseases Publication.

In: Comprehensive Diabetes Care
Editor: Joseph S. Green
ISBN: 979-8-89530-772-4

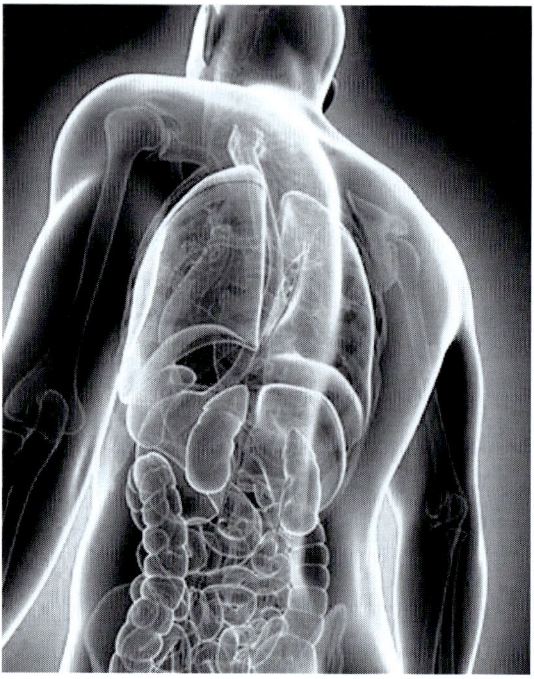

Your kidneys are located in the middle of your back, just below your rib cage.

## What Are Other Names for Diabetic Kidney Disease?

Diabetic kidney disease is also called DKD, chronic kidney disease, CKD, kidney disease of diabetes, or diabetic nephropathy.

## How Does Diabetes Cause Kidney Disease?

High blood glucose, also called blood sugar, can damage the blood vessels in your kidneys. When the blood vessels are damaged, they don't work as well. Many people with diabetes also develop high blood pressure, which can also damage your kidneys. Learn more about high blood pressure and kidney disease.

## What Increases My Chances of Developing Diabetic Kidney Disease?

Having diabetes for a longer time increases the chances that you will have kidney damage. If you have diabetes, you are more likely to develop kidney disease if your

- blood glucose is too high
- blood pressure is too high

African Americans, American Indians, and Hispanics/Latinos develop diabetes, kidney disease, and kidney failure at a higher rate than Caucasians.

You are also more likely to develop kidney disease if you have diabetes and

- smoke
- don't follow your diabetes eating plan
- eat foods high in salt
- are not active
- are overweight
- have heart disease
- have a family history of kidney failure

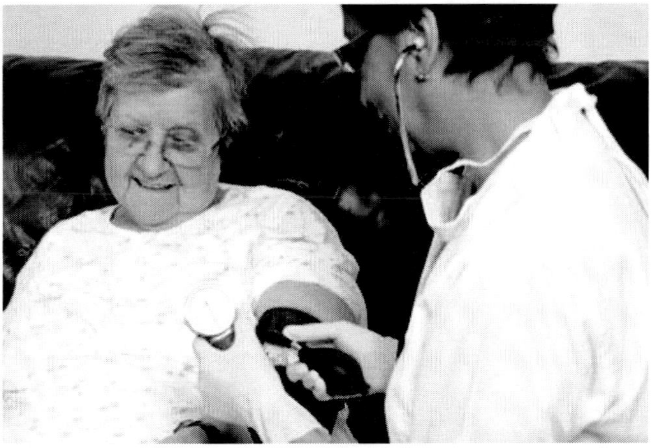

If you have diabetes, you are more likely to develop kidney disease if you have high blood pressure.

## How Can I Tell If I Have Diabetic Kidney Disease?

Most people with diabetic kidney disease do not have symptoms. The only way to know if you have diabetic kidney disease is to get your kidneys checked.

Health care professionals use blood and urine tests to check for diabetic kidney disease. Your health care professional will check your urine for albumin and will also do a blood test to see how well your kidneys are filtering your blood.

You should get tested every year for kidney disease if you

- have type 2 diabetes
- have had type 1 diabetes for more than 5 years

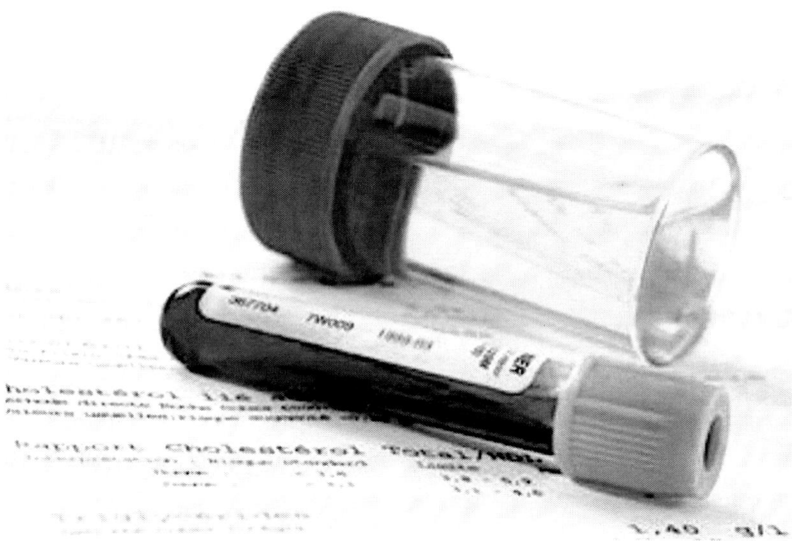

Health care professionals use blood and urine tests to check for kidney disease.

## How Can I Keep My Kidneys Healthy If I Have Diabetes?

The best way to slow or prevent diabetes-related kidney disease is to try to reach your blood glucose and blood pressure goals. Healthy lifestyle habits and taking your medicines as prescribed can help you achieve these goals and improve your health overall.

## Reach Your Blood Glucose Goals

Your health care professional will test your A1C. The A1C is a blood test that shows your average blood glucose level over the past 3 months. This is different from the blood glucose checks that you may do yourself. The higher your A1C number, the higher your blood glucose levels have been during the past 3 months.

The A1C goal for many people with diabetes is below 7 percent. Ask your health care team what your goal should be. Reaching your goal numbers will help you protect your kidneys.

To reach your A1C goal, your health care professional may ask you to check your blood glucose levels. Work with your health care team to use the results to guide decisions about food, physical activity, and medicines. Ask your health care team how often you should check your blood glucose level.

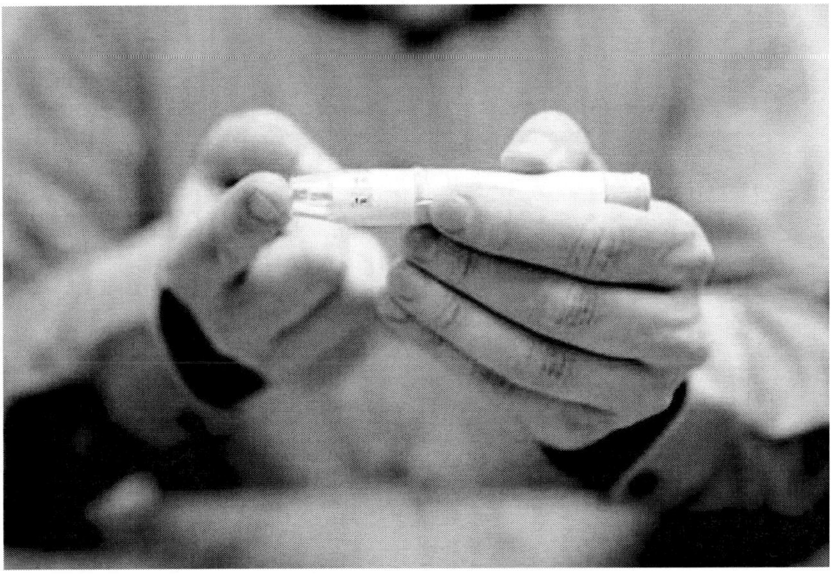

Protect your kidneys by keeping your blood glucose under control.

## Control Your Blood Pressure

Blood pressure is the force of your blood against the wall of your blood vessels. High blood pressure makes your heart work too hard. It can cause heart attack, stroke, and kidney disease.

Your health care team will also work with you to help you set and reach your blood pressure goal. The blood pressure goal for most people with diabetes is below 140/90 mm Hg. Ask your health care team what your goal should be.

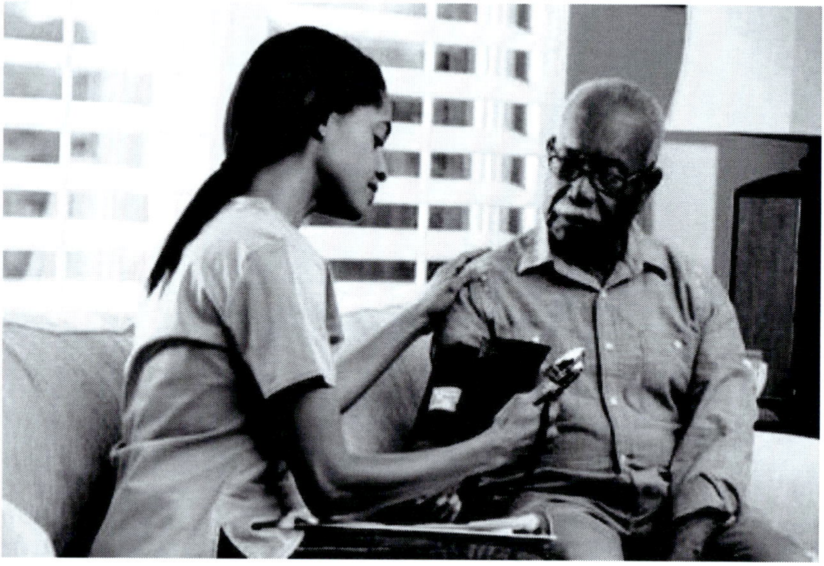

Protect your kidneys by keeping your blood pressure under control.

Medicines that lower blood pressure can also help slow kidney damage. Two types of blood pressure medicines, ACE inhibitors and ARBs, play a special role in protecting your kidneys. Each has been found to slow kidney damage in people with diabetes who have high blood pressure and DKD. The names of these medicines end in –pril or –sartan. ACE inhibitors and ARBs are not safe for women who are pregnant.

## Develop or Maintain Healthy Lifestyle Habits

Healthy lifestyle habits can help you reach your blood glucose and blood pressure goals. Following the steps below will also help you keep your kidneys healthy

- Stop smoking.
- Work with a dietitian to develop a diabetes meal plan and limit salt and sodium.
- Make physical activity part of your routine.
- Stay at or get to a healthy weight.
- Get enough sleep. Aim for 7 to 8 hours of sleep each night.

Learn more about these tips to manage diabetes.

## Take Medicines as Prescribed

Medicines may be an important part of your treatment plan. Your health care professional will prescribe medicine based on your specific needs. Medicine can help you meet your blood glucose and blood pressure goals. You may need to take more than one kind of medicine to control your blood pressure.

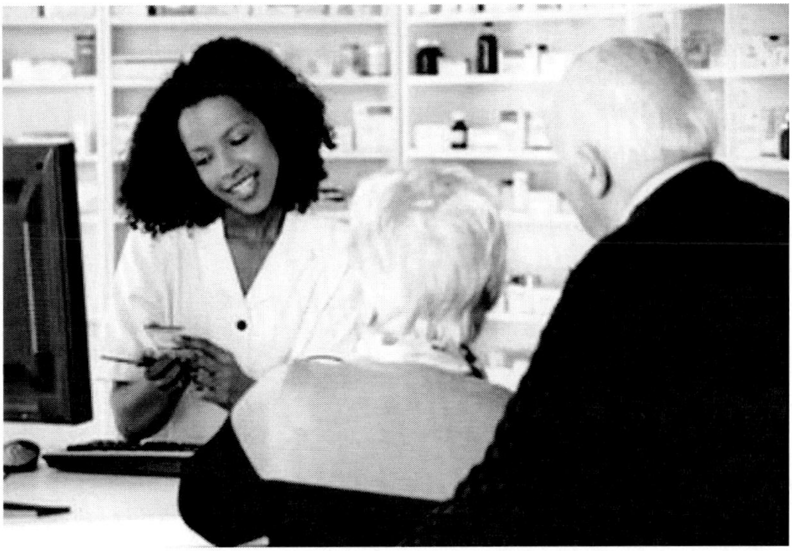

Talk to your health care professional or pharmacist about all of the medicines you take, including over-the-counter medicines.

## How Can I Cope with the Stress of Managing My Diabetes?

Managing diabetes isn't always easy. Feeling stressed, sad, or angry is common when you are living with diabetes. You may know what to do to stay healthy but may have trouble sticking with your plan over time. Long-term stress can raise your blood glucose and blood pressure, but you can learn ways to lower your stress. Try deep breathing, gardening, taking a walk, doing yoga, meditating, doing a hobby, or listening to your favorite music. Learn more about healthy ways to cope with stress *NIH external link.*

## Does Diabetic Kidney Disease Get Worse Over Time?

Kidney damage from diabetes can get worse over time. However, you can take steps to keep your kidneys healthy and help slow kidney damage to prevent or delay kidney failure. Kidney failure means that your kidneys have lost most of their ability to function—less than 15 percent of normal kidney function. However, most people with diabetes and kidney disease don't end up with kidney failure.

If your kidneys become damaged as a result of diabetes, learn how to manage kidney disease.

## Reference

[1] Centers for Disease Control and Prevention. *Chronic Kidney Disease in the United States, 2019*. Atlanta, GA: US Department of Health and Human Services. Centers for Disease Control and Prevention; 2019.

# Chapter 10

# Diabetes and Foot Problems*

## National Institute of Diabetes and Digestive and Kidney Diseases

Foot problems are common in people with diabetes. You might be afraid you'll lose a toe, foot, or leg to diabetes, or know someone who has, but you can lower your chances of having diabetes-related foot problems by taking care of your feet every day. Managing your blood glucose levels, also called blood sugar, can also help keep your feet healthy.

### How Can Diabetes Affect My Feet?

Over time, diabetes may cause nerve damage, also called diabetic neuropathy, that can cause tingling and pain, and can make you lose feeling in your feet. When you lose feeling in your feet, you may not feel a pebble inside your sock or a blister on your foot, which can lead to cuts and sores. Cuts and sores can become infected.

Diabetes also can lower the amount of blood flow in your feet. Not having enough blood flowing to your legs and feet can make it hard for a sore or an infection to heal. Sometimes, a bad infection never heals. The infection might lead to gangrene.

Gangrene and foot ulcers that do not get better with treatment can lead to an amputation of your toe, foot, or part of your leg. A surgeon may perform an amputation to prevent a bad infection from spreading to the rest of your

* This is an edited, reformatted and augmented version of National Institute of Diabetes and Digestive and Kidney Diseases Publication.

In: Comprehensive Diabetes Care
Editor: Joseph S. Green
ISBN: 979-8-89530-772-4

body, and to save your life. Good foot care is very important to prevent serious infections and gangrene.

Although rare, nerve damage from diabetes can lead to changes in the shape of your feet, such as Charcot's foot. Charcot's foot may start with redness, warmth, and swelling. Later, bones in your feet and toes can shift or break, which can cause your feet to have an odd shape, such as a "rocker bottom."

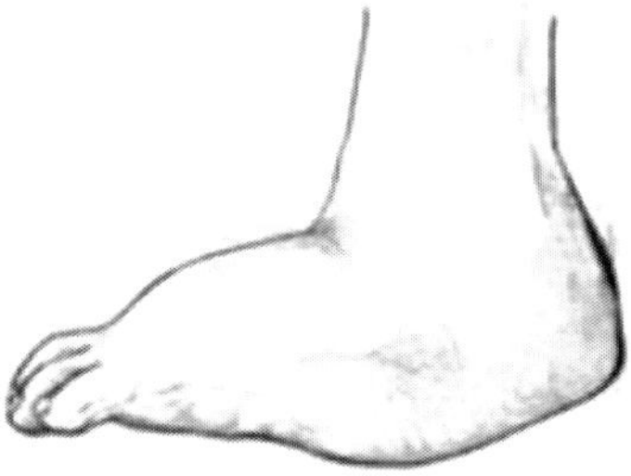

Charcot's foot can cause your feet to have an odd shape, such as a "rocker bottom."

## What Can I Do to Keep My Feet Healthy?

Work with your health care team to make a diabetes self-care plan, which is an action plan for how you will manage your diabetes. Your plan should include foot care. A foot doctor, also called a podiatrist, and other specialists may be part of your health care team.

Include these steps in your foot care plan:

## Tips to Take Care of Your Feet

- Check your feet every day.
- Wash your feet every day.
- Smooth corns and calluses gently.
- Trim your toenails straight across.
- Wear shoes and socks at all times.
- Protect your feet from hot and cold.
- Keep the blood flowing to your feet.
- Get a foot check at every health care visit.

## Check Your Feet Every Day

You may have foot problems, but feel no pain in your feet. Checking your feet each day will help you spot problems early before they get worse. A good way to remember is to check your feet each evening when you take off your shoes. Also check between your toes. If you have trouble bending over to see your feet, try using a mirror to see them, or ask someone else to look at your feet.

Look for problems such as

- cuts, sores, or red spots
- swelling or fluid-filled blisters
- ingrown toenails, in which the edge of your nail grows into your skin
- corns or calluses, which are spots of rough skin caused by too much rubbing or pressure on the same spot
- plantar warts, which are flesh-colored growths on the bottom of the feet
- athlete's foot
- warm spots

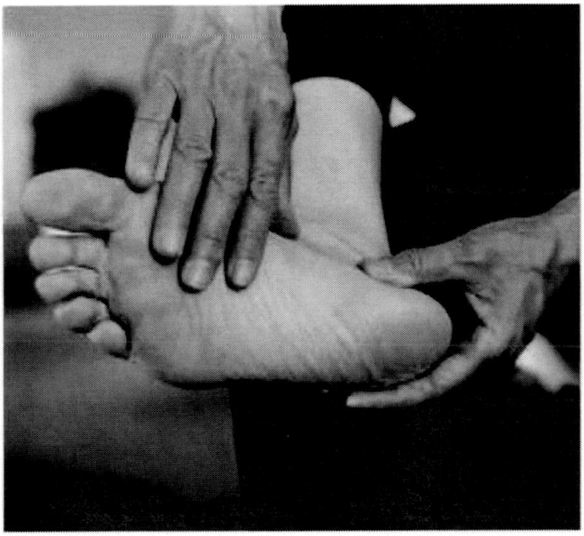

If you have certain foot problems that make it more likely you will develop a sore on your foot, your doctor may recommend taking the temperature of the skin on different parts of your feet. A "hot spot" can be the first sign that a blister or an ulcer is starting.

Cover a blister, cut, or sore with a bandage. Smooth corns and calluses as explained below.

## Wash Your Feet Every Day

Wash your feet with soap in warm, not hot, water. Test the water to make sure it is not too hot. You can use a thermometer (90° to 95° F is safe) or your elbow to test the warmth of the water. Do not soak your feet because your skin will get too dry.

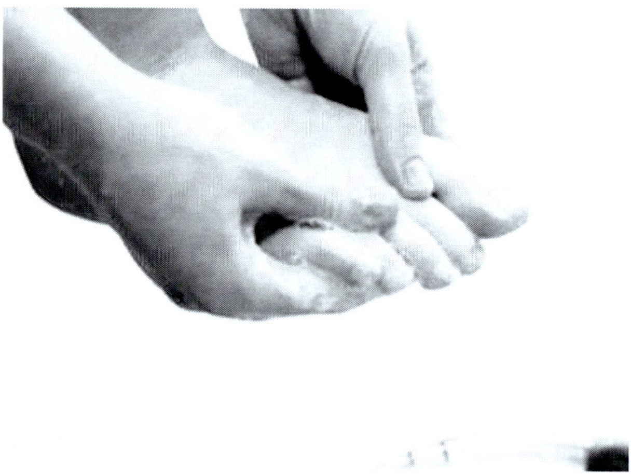

After washing and drying your feet, put talcum powder or cornstarch between your toes. Skin between the toes tends to stay moist. Powder will keep the skin dry to help prevent an infection.

## Smooth Corns and Calluses Gently

Thick patches of skin called corns or calluses can grow on the feet. If you have corns or calluses, talk with your foot doctor about the best way to care for these foot problems. If you have nerve damage, these patches can become ulcers.

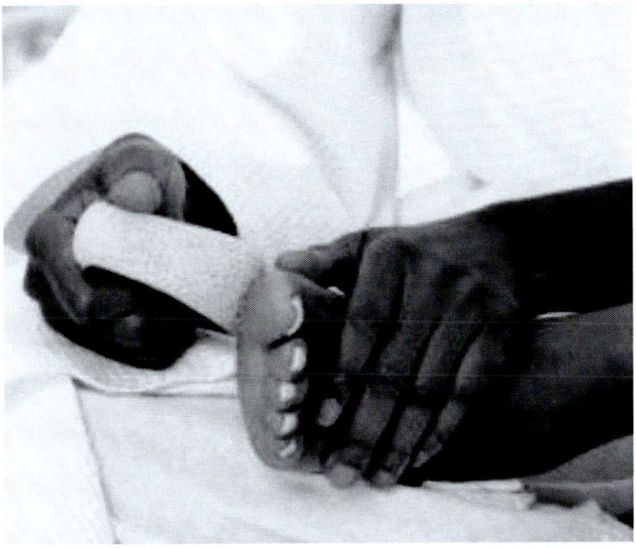

If your doctor tells you to, use a pumice stone to smooth corns and calluses after bathing or showering. A pumice stone is a type of rock used to smooth the skin. Rub gently, only in one direction, to avoid tearing the skin.

Do NOT

- cut corns and calluses
- use corn plasters, which are medicated pads
- use liquid corn and callus removers

Cutting and over-the counter corn removal products can damage your skin and cause an infection.

To keep your skin smooth and soft, rub a thin coat of lotion, cream, or petroleum jelly on the tops and bottoms of your feet. Do not put lotion or cream between your toes because moistness might cause an infection.

## Trim Your Toenails Straight Across

Trim your toenails, when needed, after you wash and dry your feet. Using toenail clippers, trim your toenails straight across. Do not cut into the corners of your toenail. Gently smooth each nail with an emery board or nonsharp nail file. Trimming this way helps prevent cutting your skin and keeps the nails from growing into your skin.

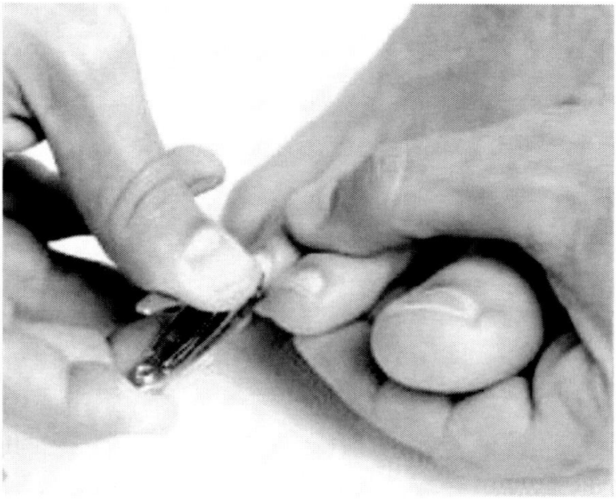

Have a foot doctor trim your toenails if

- you cannot see, feel, or reach your feet
- your toenails are thick or yellowed
- your nails curve and grow into the skin

If you want to get a pedicure at a salon, you should bring your own nail tools to prevent getting an infection. You can ask your health care provider what other steps you can take at the salon to prevent infection.

## Wear Shoes and Socks At All Times

Wear shoes and socks at all times. Do not walk barefoot or in just socks – even when you are indoors. You could step on something and hurt your feet. You may not feel any pain and may not know that you hurt yourself.

Check the inside of your shoes before putting them on, to make sure the lining is smooth and free of pebbles or other objects.

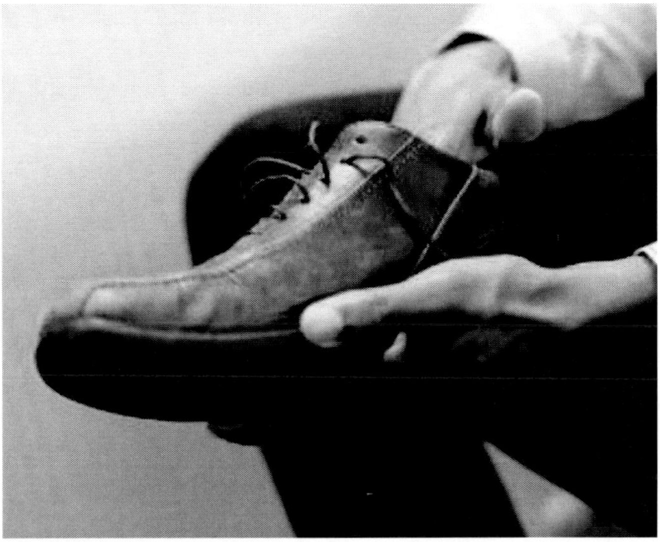

Make sure you wear socks, stockings, or nylons with your shoes to keep from getting blisters and sores. Choose clean, lightly padded socks that fit well. Socks with no seams are best.

Wear shoes that fit well and protect your feet. Here are some tips for finding the right type of shoes:

- Walking shoes and athletic shoes are good for daily wear. They support your feet and allow them to "breathe."
- Do not wear vinyl or plastic shoes, because they do not stretch or "breathe."
- When buying shoes, make sure they feel good and have enough room for your toes. Buy shoes at the end of the day, when your feet are the largest, so that you can find the best fit.
- If you have a bunion, or hammertoes, which are toes that curl under your feet, you may need extra-wide or deep shoes.1 Do not wear shoes with pointed toes or high heels, because they put too much pressure on your toes.
- If your feet have changed shape, such as from Charcot's foot, you may need special shoes or shoe inserts, called orthotics. You also may need inserts if you have bunions, hammertoes, or other foot problems.

When breaking in new shoes, only wear them for a few hours at first and then check your feet for areas of soreness.

Medicare Part B insurance External link and other health insurance programs may help pay for these special shoes or inserts. Ask your insurance plan if it covers your special shoes or inserts.

## Protect Your Feet from Hot and Cold

If you have nerve damage from diabetes, you may burn your feet and not know you did. Take the following steps to protect your feet from heat:

- Wear shoes at the beach and on hot pavement.
- Put sunscreen on the tops of your feet to prevent sunburn.
- Keep your feet away from heaters and open fires.
- Do not put a hot water bottle or heating pad on your feet.

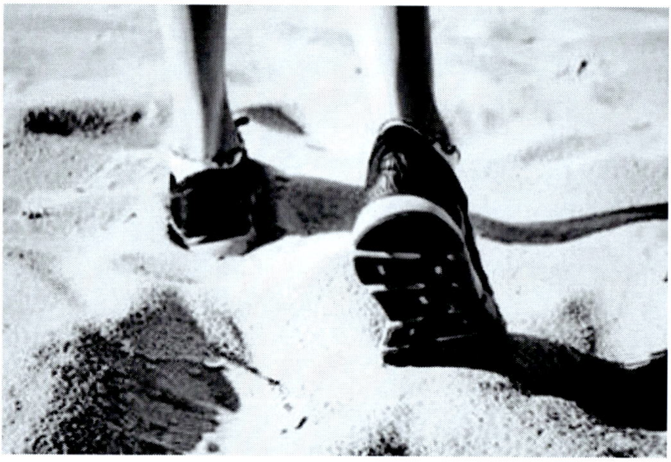

Wear socks in bed if your feet get cold. In the winter, wear lined, waterproof boots to keep your feet warm and dry.

## Keep the Blood Flowing to Your Feet

Try the following tips to improve blood flow to your feet:

- Put your feet up when you are sitting.
- Wiggle your toes for a few minutes throughout the day. Move your ankles up and down and in and out to help blood flow in your feet and legs.
- Do not wear tight socks or elastic stockings. Do not try to hold up loose socks with rubber bands.
- Be more physically active. Choose activities that are easy on your feet, such as walking, dancing, yoga or stretching, swimming, or bike riding.
- Stop smoking.

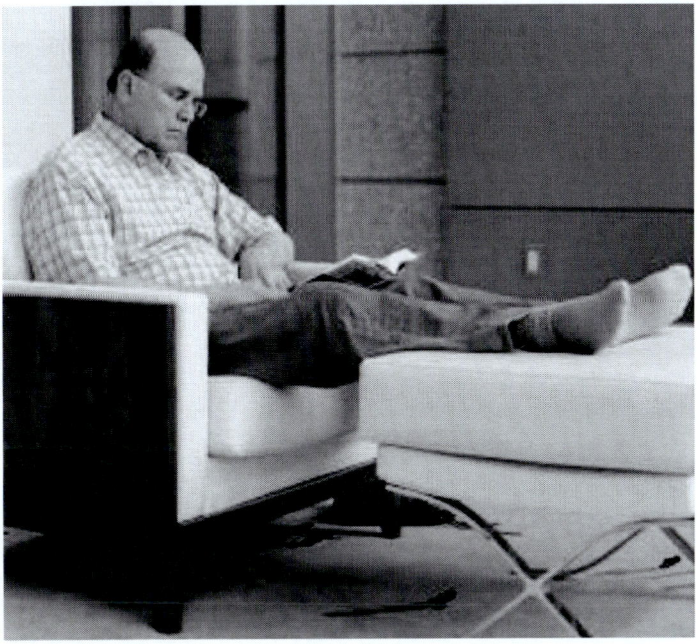

Smoking can lower the amount of blood flow to your feet. If you smoke, ask for help to stop. You can get help by calling the national quitline at 1-800-QUITNOW or 1-800-784-8669. For tips on quitting, go to SmokeFree.gov External link.

## Get a Foot Check at Every Health Care Visit

Ask your health care team to check your feet at each visit. Take off your shoes and socks when you're in the exam room so they will remember to check your feet. At least once a year, get a thorough foot exam, including a check of the feeling and pulses in your feet.

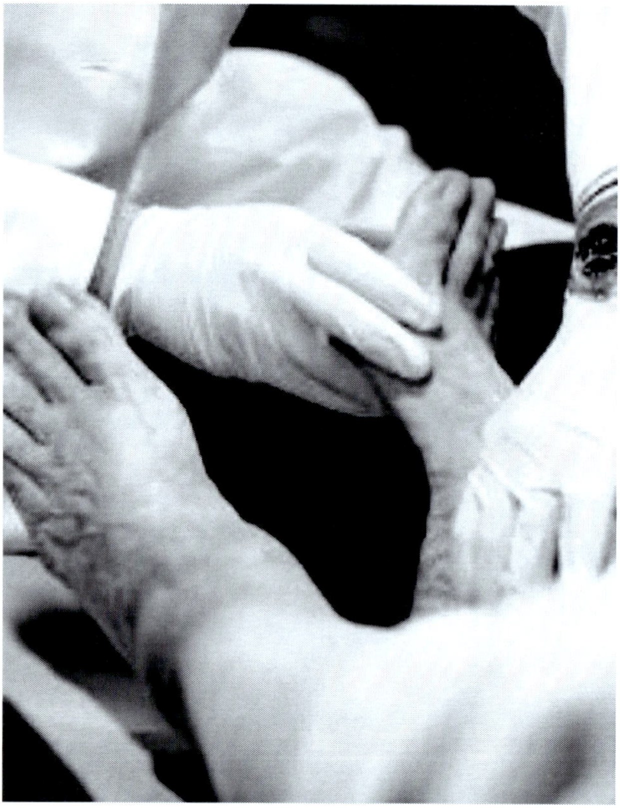

Get a thorough foot exam at each health care visit if you have

- changes in the shape of your feet
- loss of feeling in your feet
- peripheral artery disease
- had foot ulcers or an amputation in the past [1]

Ask your health care team to show you how to care for your feet.

## When Should I See My Health Care Provider About Foot Problems?

Call your health care provider right away if you have

- a cut, blister, or bruise on your foot that does not start to heal after a few days
- skin on your foot that becomes red, warm, or painful—signs of a possiblc infcction
- a callus with dried blood inside of it,which often can be the first sign of a wound under the callus
- a foot infection that becomes black and smelly—signs you might have gangrene

Ask your provider to refer you to a foot doctor, or podiatrist, if needed.

## Clinical Trials

The National Institute of Diabetes and Digestive and Kidney Diseases (NIDDK) and other components of the National Institutes of Health (NIH) conduct and support research into many diseases and conditions.

## What Are Clinical Trials, and Are They Right for You?

Clinical trials are part of clinical research and at the heart of all medical advances. Clinical trials look at new ways to prevent, detect, or treat disease. Researchers also use clinical trials to look at other aspects of care, such as improving the quality of life for people with chronic illnesses. Find out if clinical trials are right for you *NIH external link*.

## What Clinical Trials Are Open?

Clinical trials that are currently open and are recruiting can be viewed at www.ClinicalTrials.gov *NIH external link*.

## Reference

[1] American Diabetes Association. Microvascular complications and foot care. *Diabetes Care.* 2016;39(Suppl. 1):S78.

# Chapter 11

# Diabetic Eye Disease*


## National Institute of Diabetes and Digestive and Kidney Diseases


## What Is Diabetic Eye Disease?

Diabetic eye disease is a group of eye problems that can affect people with diabetes. These conditions include diabetic retinopathy, diabetic macular edema, cataracts, and glaucoma.

Over time, diabetes can cause damage to your eyes that can lead to poor vision or even blindness. But you can take steps to prevent diabetic eye disease, or keep it from getting worse, by taking care of your diabetes.

The best ways to manage your diabetes and keep your eyes healthy are to

- manage your blood glucose, blood pressure, and cholesterol, sometimes called the diabetes ABCs
- If you smoke, get help to quit smoking External link
- have a dilated eye exam once a year

* This is an edited, reformatted and augmented version of National Institute of Diabetes and Digestive and Kidney Diseases Publication.


In: Comprehensive Diabetes Care
Editor: Joseph S. Green
ISBN: 979-8-89530-772-4

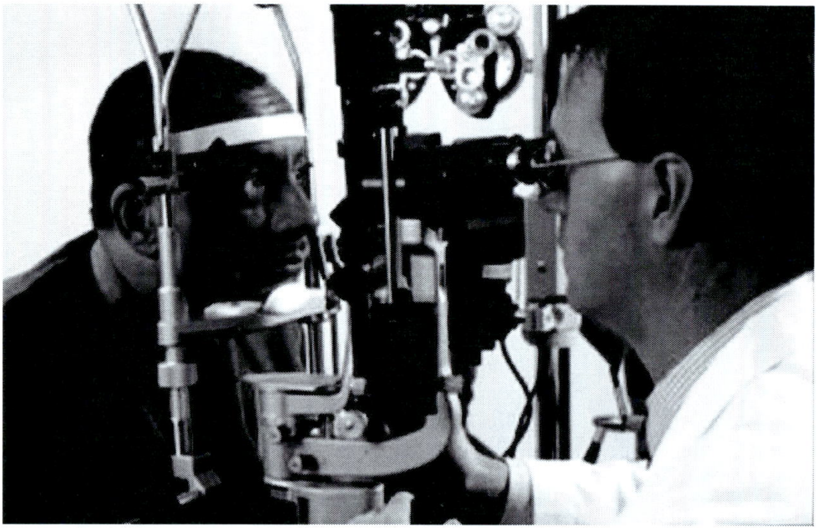

Photo courtesy of the National Eye Institute, NIH.

Your eyes may seem fine, but having a full, dilated eye exam is the only way to know for sure.

Often, there are no warning signs of diabetic eye disease or vision loss when damage first develops. A full, dilated eye exam helps your doctor find and treat eye problems early—often before much vision loss can occur.

## How Does Diabetes Affect My Eyes?

Diabetes affects your eyes when your blood glucose, also called blood sugar, is too high.

*In the short term,* you are not likely to have vision loss from high blood glucose. People sometimes have blurry vision for a few days or weeks when they're changing their diabetes care plan or medicines. High glucose can change fluid levels or cause swelling in the tissues of your eyes *NIH external link* that help you to focus, causing blurred vision. This type of blurry vision is temporary and goes away when your glucose level gets closer to normal.

*If your blood glucose stays high over time,* it can damage the tiny blood vessels in the back of your eyes. This damage can begin during prediabetes, when blood glucose is higher than normal, but not high enough for you to be diagnosed with diabetes. Damaged blood vessels may leak fluid and cause swelling. New, weak blood vessels may also begin to grow. These blood vessels can bleed into the middle part of the eye, lead to scarring, or cause dangerously high pressure inside your eye.

Most serious diabctic eye diseases begin with blood vessel problems. The four eye diseases that can threaten your sight are:

## Diabetic Retinopathy

The retina NIH external link is the inner lining at the back of each eye. The retina senses light and turns it into signals that your brain decodes, so you can see the world around you. Damaged blood vessels can harm the retina, causing a disease called diabetic retinopathy.

In early diabetic retinopathy, blood vessels can weaken, bulge, or leak into the retina. This stage is called nonproliferative diabetic retinopathy.

If the disease gets worse, some blood vessels close off, which causes new blood vessels to grow, or proliferate, on the surface of the retina. This stage is called proliferative diabetic retinopathy. These abnormal new blood vessels can lead to serious vision problems.

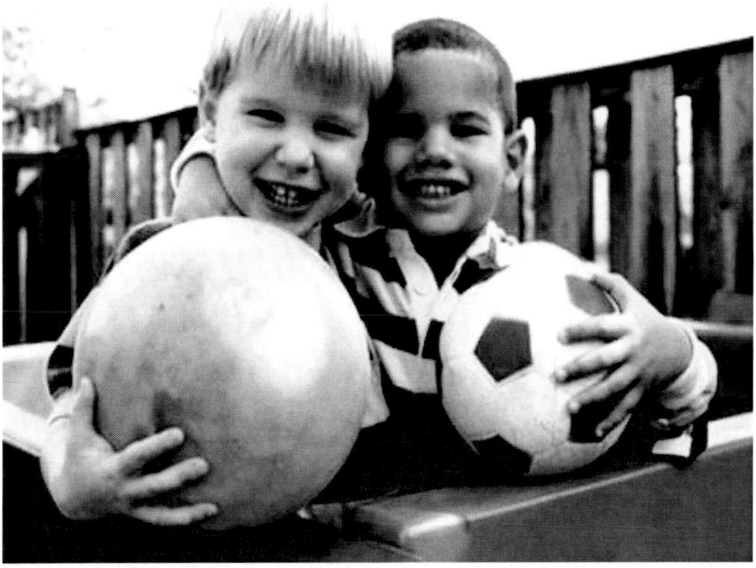

Photo courtesy of the National Eye Institute, NIH.

Normal vision of two boys playing.

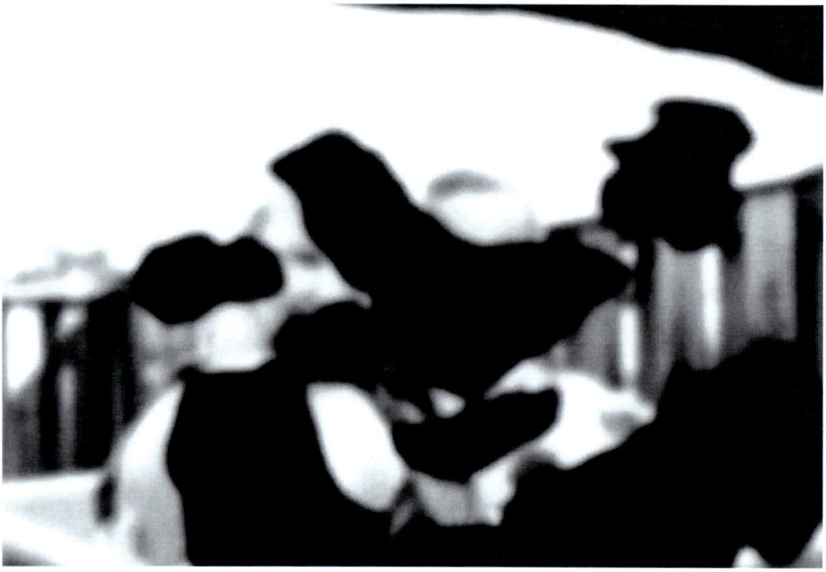

Photo courtesy of the National Eye Institute, NIH.

Same scene, as viewed by a person with diabetic retinopathy.

## Diabetic Macular Edema

The part of your retina that you need for reading, driving, and seeing faces is called the macula. Diabetes can lead to swelling in the macula, which is called diabetic macular edema. Over time, this disease can destroy the sharp vision in this part of the eye, leading to partial vision loss or blindness. Macular edema usually develops in people who already have other signs of diabetic retinopathy.

## Glaucoma

Glaucoma is a group of eye diseases that can damage the optic nerve—the bundle of nerves that connects the eye to the brain. Diabetes doubles the chances of having glaucoma, which can lead to vision loss and blindness if not treated early.

Symptoms depend on which type of glaucoma you have. Learn more about glaucoma *NIH external link*.

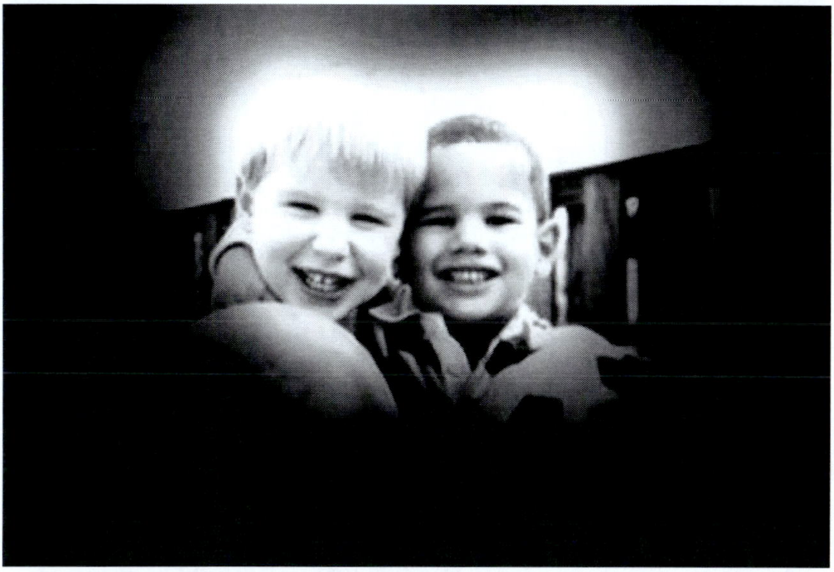

Photo courtesy of the National Eye Institute, NIH.

People with glaucoma slowly lose side vision.

## Cataracts

The lenses within our eyes are clear structures that help provide sharp vision—but they tend to become cloudy as we age. People with diabetes are more likely to develop cloudy lenses, called cataracts. People with diabetes can develop cataracts at an earlier age than people without diabetes. Researchers think that high glucose levels cause deposits to build up in the lenses of your eyes.

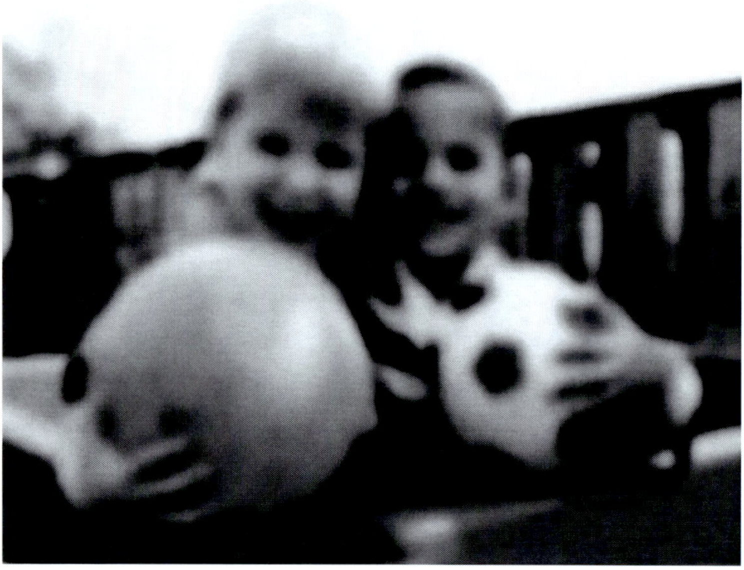

Photo courtesy of the National Eye Institute, NIH.

Cloudy vision and faded colors are symptoms of cataracts.

## How Common Is Diabetic Eye Disease?

### Diabetic Retinopathy

About one in three people with diabetes who are older than age 40 already have some signs of diabetic retinopathy [1]. Diabetic retinopathy is the most common cause of vision loss in people with diabetes. Each person's outlook for the future, however, depends in large part on regular care. Finding and treating diabetic retinopathy early can reduce the risk of blindness by 95 percent.

### Glaucoma and Cataracts

Your chances of developing glaucoma or cataracts are about twice that of someone without diabetes.

## Who Is More Likely to Develop Diabetic Eye Disease?

Anyone with diabetes can develop diabetic eye disease. Your risk is greater with

- high blood glucose that is not treated
- high blood pressure that is not treated

High blood cholesterol and smoking may also raise your risk for diabetic eye disease.

Some groups are affected more than others. African Americans, American Indians and Alaska Natives, Hispanics/Latinos, Pacific Islanders, and older adults are at greater risk of losing vision or going blind from diabetes.

If you have diabetes and become pregnant, you can develop eye problems very quickly during your pregnancy. If you already have some diabetic retinopathy, it can get worse during pregnancy. Changes that help your body support a growing baby may put stress on the blood vessels in your eyes. Your health care team will suggest regular eye exams during pregnancy to catch and treat problems early and protect your vision.

Diabetes that occurs only during pregnancy, called gestational diabetes, does not usually cause eye problems. Researchers aren't sure why this is the case.

Your chances of developing diabetic eye disease increase the longer you have diabetes.

## What Are the Symptoms of Diabetic Eye Disease?

Often there are no early symptoms of diabetic eye disease. You may have no pain and no change in your vision as damage begins to grow inside your eyes, particularly with diabetic retinopathy.

When symptoms do occur, they may include

- blurry or wavy vision
- frequently changing vision—sometimes from day to day
- dark areas or vision loss
- poor color vision
- spots or dark strings (also called floaters)

- flashes of light

Talk with your eye doctor if you have any of these symptoms.

## When Should I See a Doctor Right Away?

Call a doctor right away if you notice sudden changes to your vision, including flashes of light or many more spots (floaters) than usual. You also should see a doctor right away if it looks like a curtain is pulled over your eyes. These changes in your sight can be symptoms of a detached retina NIH external link, which is a medical emergency.

## How Do Doctors Diagnose Eye Problems from Diabetes?

Having a full, dilated eye exam is the best way to check for eye problems from diabetes. Your doctor will place drops in your eyes to widen your pupils. This allows the doctor to examine a larger area at the back of each eye, using a special magnifying lens. Your vision will be blurry for a few hours after a dilated exam.

Your doctor will also

- test your vision
- measure the pressure in your eyes

Your doctor may suggest other tests, too, depending on your health history.

Most people with diabetes should see an eye care professional once a year for a complete eye exam. Your own health care team may suggest a different plan, based on your type of diabetes and the time since you were first diagnosed.

## Eye Exam Guidelines for Diabetes [2, 3, 4]:

- Type 1: Yearly eye exams should start within 5 years of diagnosis.
- Type 2: Yearly eye exams should start right after diagnosis.

- Pregnancy: Women with type 1 and type 2 diabetes need an eye exam before pregnancy or within the first 3 months. Your doctor may want you to repeat the exam later in your pregnancy and until your baby is 1 year old.

Women who develop gestational diabetes don't usually need an eye exam because they don't develop diabetic eye disease during pregnancy. If you have any questions, ask your doctor.

## How Do Doctors Treat Diabetic Eye Disease?

Your doctor may recommend having eye exams more often than once a year, along with management of your diabetes. This means managing your diabetes ABCs, which include your A1c, blood pressure, and cholesterol; and quitting smoking. Ask your health care team what you can do to reach your goals.

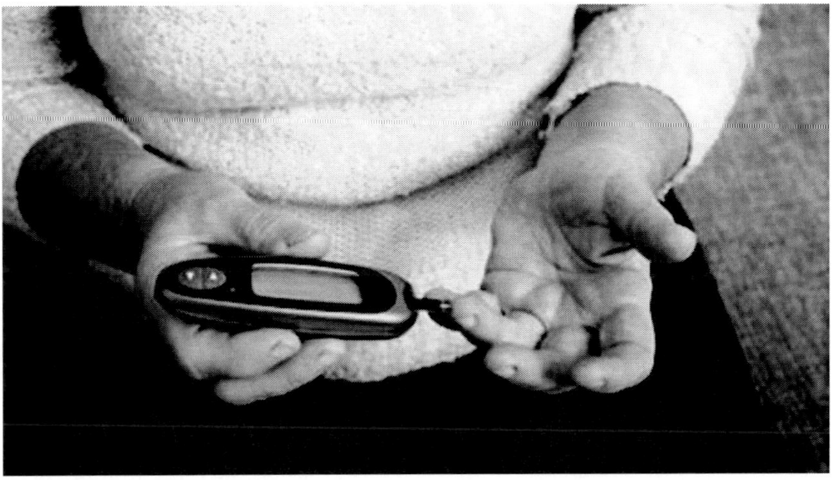

Management of blood glucose can help prevent diabetic eye disease and keep it from getting worse.

Doctors may treat advanced eye problems NIH external link with medicine, laser treatments, surgery, or a combination of these options.

### Medicine

Your doctor may treat your eyes with anti-VEGF medicine, such as aflibercept, bevacizumab, or ranibizumab. These medicines block the growth of abnormal blood vessels in the eye. Anti-VEGF medicines can also stop fluid leaks, which can help treat diabetic macular edema.

The doctor will inject an anti-VEGF medicine into your eyes during office visits. You'll have several treatments during the first few months, then fewer treatments after you finish the first round of therapy. Your doctor will use medicine to numb your eyes so you don't feel pain. The needle is about the thickness of a human hair.

Anti-VEGF treatments can stop further vision loss and may improve vision in some people.

### Laser Treatment

Laser treatment, also called photocoagulation, creates tiny burns inside the eye with a beam of light. This method treats leaky blood vessels and extra fluid, called edema. Your doctor usually provides this treatment during several office visits, using medicine to numb your eyes. Laser treatment can keep eye disease from getting worse, which is important to prevent vision loss or blindness. But laser treatment is less likely to bring back vision you've already lost compared with anti-VEGF medicines.

There are two types of laser treatment NIH external link:

- Focal/grid laser treatment works on a small area of the retina to treat diabetic macular edema.
- Scatter laser treatment, also called panretinal photocoagulation (PRP), covers a larger area of the retina. This method treats the growth of abnormal blood vessels, called proliferative diabetic retinopathy.

### Vitrectomy

Vitrectomy is a surgery to remove the clear gel that fills the center of the eye, called the vitreous gel. The procedure treats problems with severe bleeding or scar tissue caused by proliferative diabetic retinopathy. Scar tissue can force the retina to peel away from the tissue beneath it, like wallpaper peeling away from a wall. A retina that comes completely loose, or detaches, can cause blindness.

During vitrectomy, a clear salt solution is gently pumped into the eye to maintain eye pressure during surgery and to replace the removed vitreous. Vitrectomy is done in a surgery center or hospital with pain medicine.

### Cataract Lens Surgery

In a surgery center or hospital visit, your doctor can remove the cloudy lens in your eye, where the cataract has grown, and replace it with an artificial lens. People who have cataract surgery generally have better vision afterward. After your eye heals, you may need a new prescription for your glasses. Your vision following cataract surgery may also depend on treating any damage from diabetic retinopathy or macular edema.

## What Can I Do to Protect My Eyes?

To prevent diabetic eye disease, or to keep it from getting worse, manage your diabetes ABCs: your A1c, blood pressure, and cholesterol; and quit smoking if you smoke. Read more information on how to manage diabetes.

Also, have a dilated eye exam *NIH external link* at least once a year—or more often if recommended by your eye care professional. These actions are powerful ways to protect the health of your eyes—and can prevent blindness.

The sooner you work to manage your diabetes and other health conditions, the better. And, even if you've struggled in the past to manage your health, taking better care of yourself now can protect your eyes for the future. It's never too late to begin.

## What If I Already Have Some Vision Loss from Diabetes?

Ask your eye care professional to help you find a low vision NIH external link and rehabilitation clinic. Special eye care professionals can help you manage vision loss that cannot be corrected with glasses, contact lenses, medicine, or surgery. Special devices and training may help you make the most of your remaining vision so that you can continue to be active, enjoy hobbies, visit friends and family members, and live without help from others.

## References

[1] Centers for Disease Control and Prevention. National Diabetes Statistics Report: Estimates of Diabetes and Its Burden in the United States, 2014. Atlanta, GA: *U.S. Department of Health and Human Services;* 2014.

[2] Diabetic retinopathy preferred practice pattern guidelines. American Academy of Ophthalmology website. https://www.aao.org/preferred-practice-pattern/diabetic-retinopathy-ppp External link. Updated January 2016. Accessed June 2, 2017.

[3] Fraser CE, D'Amico DJ. Diabetic retinopathy: prevention and treatment. UpToDate website. https://www.uptodate.com/contents/diabetic-retinopathy-prevention-and-treatment External link. September 28, 2016. Accessed June 2, 2017.

[4] American Diabetes Association. Standards of medical care in diabetes—2016 abridged for primary care providers. *Clinical Diabetes.* 2016 Jan;34(1):3–21.

# Chapter 12

# Diabetic Eye Disease: Five Things You Should Know About Diabetic Eye Disease*


## National Eye Institute


Did you know that diabetes can cause eye disease? If left untreated, it can cause vision loss or even blindness. To help you keep your vision healthy, here are five things the National Eye Institute (NEI) would like you to know about diabetic eye disease:

## 1. A Group of Eye Problems

People with diabetes may face several eye problems as a complication of this disease. They include cataract, glaucoma, and diabetic retinopathy, which is the leading cause of blindness in American adults age 20–74.

## 2. No Symptoms, No Pain

In its early stages, diabetic retinopathy has no symptoms. A person may not notice vision changes until the disease advances. Blurred vision may occur when the macula swells from the leaking fluid (called macular edema). If new vessels have grown on the surface of the retina, they can bleed into the eye, blocking vision.

* This is an edited, reformatted and augmented version of A program of the National Institutes of Health, National Yey Institute Publication.


In: Comprehensive Diabetes Care
Editor: Joseph S. Green
ISBN: 979-8-89530-772-4

## 3. Have Diabetes? You Are at Risk

Anyone with diabetes is at risk of getting diabetic retinopathy. The longer someone has diabetes, the more likely he or she will get this eye disease.

In fact, between 40 and 45 percent of those with diagnosed diabetes have some degree of diabetic retinopathy.

## 4. Stay on TRACK

That is: Take your medications as prescribed by your doctor; Reach and maintain a healthy weight; Add more physical activity to your daily routine; Control your ABC's—A1C, blood pressure, and cholesterol levels; and Kick the smoking habit.

## 5. Get a Dilated Eye Exam

### Video

This video describes what the doctor sees when examining the retina (the light-sensitive tissue at the back of the eye), macula (the part of the retina needed for sharp, central vision), and optic nerve (which connects the retina to the brain).

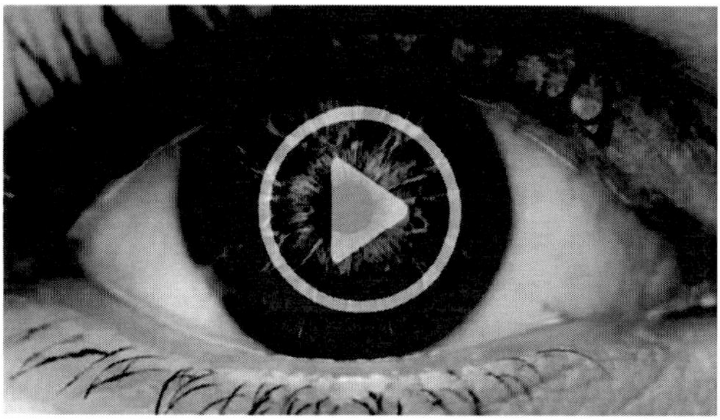

To learn more, visit http://www.nei.nih.gov/diabetes.

Chapter 13

# Start the Conversation About Diabetes: Educating Older Adults About Diabetic Eye Disease*

## National Eye Institute

Diabetes is an epidemic in the United States. In the past 30 years, the number of adults diagnosed with diabetes has increased by more than 150 percent.[1] Diabetes can cause many health problems, including vision loss and blindness. The longer a person has diabetes, the higher his or her risk is of getting diabetic eye disease, yet half of all people with diabetes don't get annual comprehensive dilated eye exams. Start the conversation about diabetic eye disease so you can help people with diabetes protect their sight.

## What Is Diabetic Eye Disease?

Diabetic eye disease refers to a group of eye problems people with diabetes may face as a complication of this disease, which can lead to vision loss and blindness. These include—

- *Cataract:* Clouding of the lens of the eye

* This is an edited, reformatted and augmented version of a Tip Sheet of a Program of the National Institutes of Health, National Yey Institute Publication.

[1] Centers for Disease Control and Prevention. Crude and Age-Adjusted Percentage of Civilian, Noninstitutionalized Adults with Diagnosed Diabetes, United States, 1980–2011. Atlanta, GA: U.S. Department of Health and Human Services; 2013. Available at http://www.cdc.gov/diabetes/statistics/prev/national/figageadult.htm.

In: Comprehensive Diabetes Care
Editor: Joseph S. Green
ISBN: 979-8-89530-772-4

- *Diabetic retinopathy:* Damage to the blood vessels in the retina, the light-sensitive tissue in the back of the eye
- *Glaucoma:* Increase in fluid pressure inside the eye that leads to optic nerve damage and loss of vision

To help prevent vision loss and blindness, it's important for people with diabetes to have a comprehensive dilated eye exam at least once a year to detect diabetic eye disease early and to keep their diabetes under control.

## What Are the Symptoms of Diabetic Eye Disease?

Diabetic retinopathy is the most common of the diabetic eye diseases. It often has no early symptoms; however, less than 10 percent of adults ages 65 and older in the United States are aware of this.[2] It is vital they be informed that diabetic retinopathy can cause vision loss that usually cannot be restored but that vision loss can be prevented or minimized with early detection, timely treatment, and appropriate follow-up care.

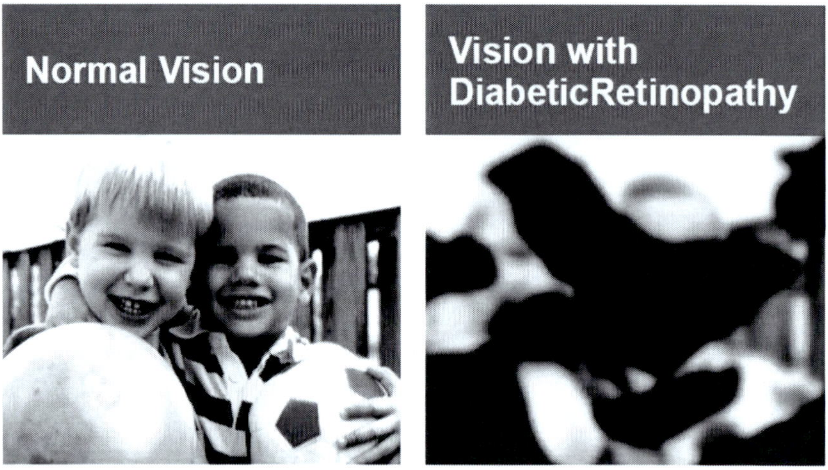


[2] National Eye Health Education Program et al. *2005 Survey of Public Knowledge, Attitudes, and Practices Related to Eye Health and Disease*, 2005. Bethesda, MD: National Eye Institute.

Tip Box

To help older adults reduce their risk of vision loss and blindness, encourage them to get a comprehensive dilated eye exam every year and to control their diabetes by—

- Taking their medications.
- Reaching and maintaining a healthy weight.
- Adding physical activity to their daily routine.
- Controlling their blood sugar, blood pressure, and cholesterol.
- Kicking the smoking habit.

## Older Adults, Diabetes, and Diabetic Retinopathy

Vision loss and blindness are not a normal part of the aging process, however, as people with diabetes age, they are at an increased risk for eye disease, especially diabetic retinopathy. More than 11 million, or more than 25 percent, of all people 65 years of age and older have diabetes,[3] and more than 3 million adults ages 65 and older have diabetic retinopathy.[4]

## Older Adults and Health Care

Many older adults have concerns about paying for eye exams, and some treat eye problems using natural medicine and home remedies.[5] Help protect the sight of older adults by sharing science-based information with them.

## What You Can Do

As a health or community-based professional, you can guide, motivate, and encourage older adults with diabetes to protect their vision. Please visit the National Eye Institute (NEI) Publications Catalog (https://catalog.nei.

[3] Centers for Disease Control and Prevention. *National Diabetes Statistics Report: Estimates of Diabetes and Its Burden in the United States, 2014*. Atlanta, GA: U.S. Department of Health and Human Services; 2014. Available at http://www.cdc.gov/diabetes/pubs/ statsreport14 /national-diabetes-report-web.pdf.

[4] National Eye Institute. *2010 U.S. Prevalent Cases of Diabetic Retinopathy (in Thousands) by Age, Race/Ethnicity*, 2012. Available at https://www.nei.nih.gov/eyedata/diabetic.asp#3.

[5] National Eye Health Education Program. Summary Topline Report #17: Older Adults Combined, 2011. Unpublished. Bethesda, MD: National Eye Institute.

nih.gov/) and download diabetic eye disease resources (available in English and Spanish) for your discussions. These resources can help you raise awareness about how older adults with diabetes can protect their sight.

Help the National Eye Health Education Program (NEHEP) spread the word:

- Discuss the relationship between diabetes and vision with your patients or those you serve.
- Have copies of NEHEP resources available and share them in your office.
- Post or tweet the following call to action on your Facebook and Twitter sites: Everyone with diabetes needs to get a comprehensive dilated eye exam at least once a year.
- Host a health-related event at your location, at a local health fair or senior center, or in a place of worship, and speak about diabetic eye disease and the importance of healthy vision. Remind older adults that people with diabetes need to have a comprehensive dilated eye exam at least once a year.
- Share information about financial aid for eye care.
- Take extra time to answer questions during health appointments (if you are a healthcare provider) and make sure patients understand their role in maintaining healthy vision. If a caregiver or family member is with them, please make sure that he or she understands the information you provide.

## Diabetic Eye Disease Resources

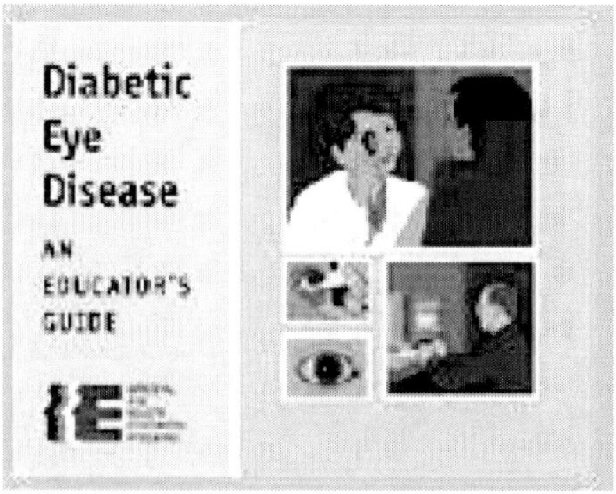

- *Diabetic Eye Disease:* An Educator's Guide—This patient education tool for health professionals and community-based educators is a desktop flipchart, with text and illustrations to help guide discussions with people who have diabetes.

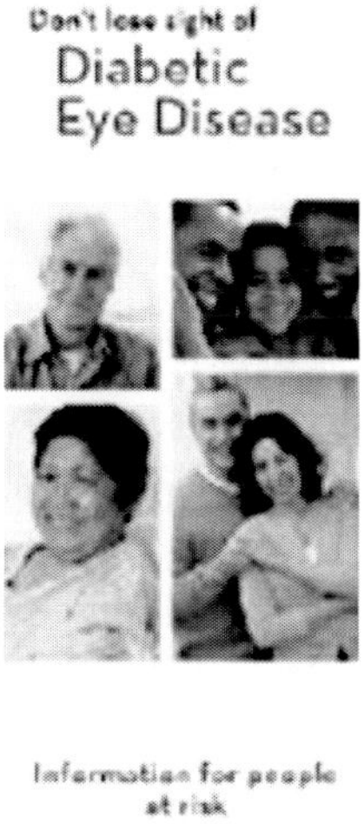


- *Don't Lose Sight of Diabetic Eye Disease*—This brochure provides information about diabetic eye disease and what people can do to prevent vision loss.

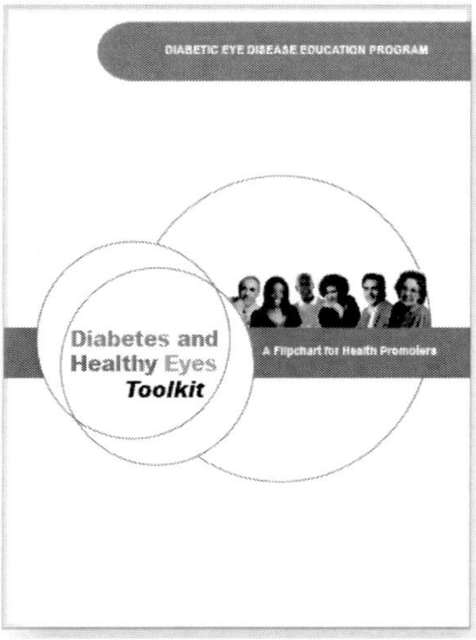

- *Diabetes and Healthy Eyes Toolkit*—This educational toolkit provides community health workers and health promoters with information and tools to help them educate people about diabetic eye disease in small group settings.

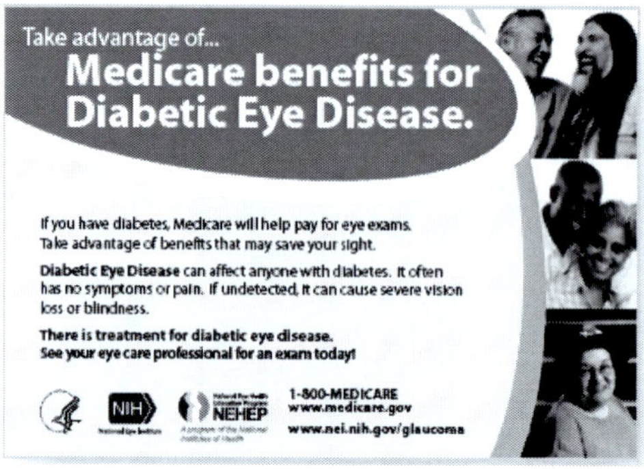
Take advantage of...
Medicare benefits for Diabetic Eye Disease.
If you have diabetes, Medicare will help pay for eye exams. Take advantage of benefits that may save your sight.
Diabetic Eye Disease can affect anyone with diabetes. It often has no symptoms or pain. If undetected, it can cause severe vision loss or blindness.
There is treatment for diabetic eye disease. See your eye care professional for an exam today!
NIH
NEHEP
1-800-MEDICARE
www.medicare.gov
www.nei.nih.gov/glaucoma

- *Medicare Benefit Card*—This card promotes the glaucoma and diabetic eye disease benefit under Medicare and describes eligibility requirements.

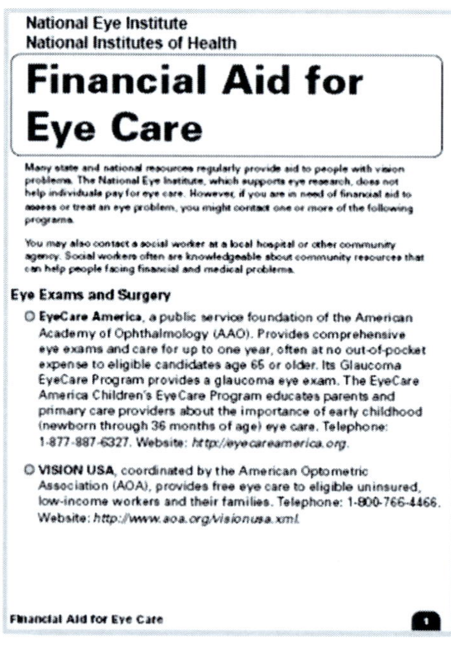

National Eye Institute
National Institutes of Health

**Financial Aid for Eye Care**

Many state and national resources regularly provide aid to people with vision problems. The National Eye Institute, which supports eye research, does not help individuals pay for eye care. However, if you are in need of financial aid to assess or treat an eye problem, you might contact one or more of the following programs.

You may also contact a social worker at a local hospital or other community agency. Social workers often are knowledgeable about community resources that can help people facing financial and medical problems.

**Eye Exams and Surgery**

- **EyeCare America**, a public service foundation of the American Academy of Ophthalmology (AAO). Provides comprehensive eye exams and care for up to one year, often at no out-of-pocket expense to eligible candidates age 65 or older. Its Glaucoma EyeCare Program provides a glaucoma eye exam. The EyeCare America Children's EyeCare Program educates parents and primary care providers about the importance of early childhood (newborn through 36 months of age) eye care. Telephone: 1-877-887-6327. Website: *http://eyecareamerica.org*.
- **VISION USA**, coordinated by the American Optometric Association (AOA), provides free eye care to eligible uninsured, low-income workers and their families. Telephone: 1-800-766-4466. Website: *http://www.aoa.org/visionusa.xml*.

Financial Aid for Eye Care 1

- *Financial Aid for Eye Care*—This handout lists state and national resources that regularly provide aid to people with vision problems.

## Other Diabetic Eye Disease Resources

NEHEP provides additional resources you can use year-round on your website, in your newsletter,

or with any other educational or outreach efforts. Check these out at www.nei.nih.gov/nehep/ programs/diabeticeyedisease

- Diabetic eye disease education website
- Drop-in articles
- Infocards
- Print public service announcements
- Social media messages
- Videos and animations
- Web banners

## Join us!

Together, we can make a difference. We look forward to working with you to help people with diabetes protect their sight.

For more information on diabetic eye disease, visit www.nei.nih.gov/ diabetes or call NEI at 301–496–5248.

# Chapter 14

# People with Diabetes Can Prevent Vision Loss*

## National Eye Institute

You can't feel it. You can't see it—until it's too late. Diabetic retinopathy, the most common form of diabetic eye disease, is the leading cause of blindness in adults age 20–74. It occurs when diabetes damages blood vessels in the retina.

| Did You Know? |
|---|
| • Everyone with diabetes is at risk for diabetic retinopathy.<br>• There are no early symptoms.<br>• A dilated eye exam can detect eye disease before vision loss occurs.<br>• Don't wait until you notice an eye problem to have an exam. |

Diabetic retinopathy affects 7.7 million Americans, and that number is projected to increase to more than 14.6 million people by 2030.

The longer a person has diabetes, the greater the risk for diabetic eye disease. Once vision is lost, it often cannot be restored.

People with diabetes should have a comprehensive dilated eye exam at least once a year to help protect their sight.

Keeping diabetes in control is key to slowing the progression of vision complications like diabetic retinopathy. There are important steps people with diabetes can take to keep their health on TRACK:

* This is an edited, reformatted and augmented version of the National Institutes of Health, National Eye Institute Publication.

In: Comprehensive Diabetes Care
Editor: Joseph S. Green
ISBN: 979-8-89530-772-4

- Take your medications as prescribed by your doctor.
- Reach and maintain a healthy weight.
- Add physical activity to your daily routine.
- Control your ABC's—A1C, blood pressure, and cholesterol levels.
- Kick the smoking habit.

Early detection, timely treatment, and appropriate follow-up care can reduce a person's risk for severe vision loss from diabetic eye disease by 95 percent.

Dr. Paul Sieving, director of the National Eye Institute (NEI), says, "Only about half of all people with diabetes get an annual comprehensive dilated eye exam, which is essential for detecting diabetic eye disease early, when it is most treatable. Newer and better treatments are available for the first time in decades, making early detection even more important."

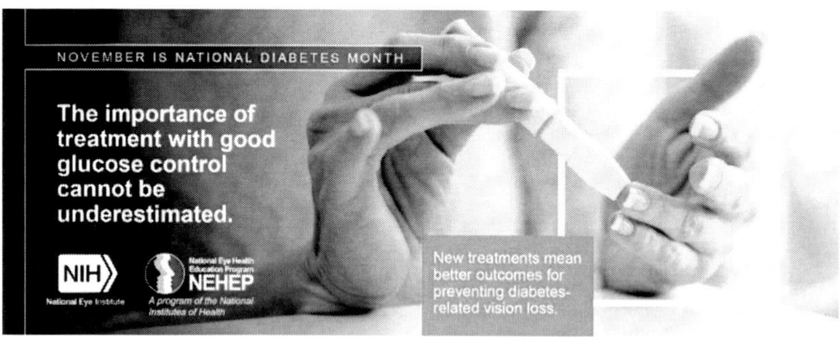


With no early symptoms, diabetic eye disease—a group of conditions including cataract, glaucoma, and diabetic retinopathy—can affect anyone with type 1 or type 2 diabetes. African Americans, American Indians/Alaska Natives, and Hispanics/Latinos are at higher risk for losing vision or going blind from diabetes.

"More than ever, it's important for people with diabetes to have a comprehensive dilated eye exam at least once a year. New treatments are being developed all the time, and we are learning that different treatments may work best for different patients. What hasn't changed is that early treatment is always better," says Dr. Suber Huang, chair of the Diabetic Eye Disease Subcommittee for NEI's National Eye Health Education Program (NEHEP) and member of the NEI-funded Diabetic Retinopathy Clinical Research

Network (DRCR.net). "There has never been a more hopeful time in the treatment of diabetic retinopathy," he adds.

**Projected Increase of Diabetic Retinopathy in the United States, by Ethnicity**

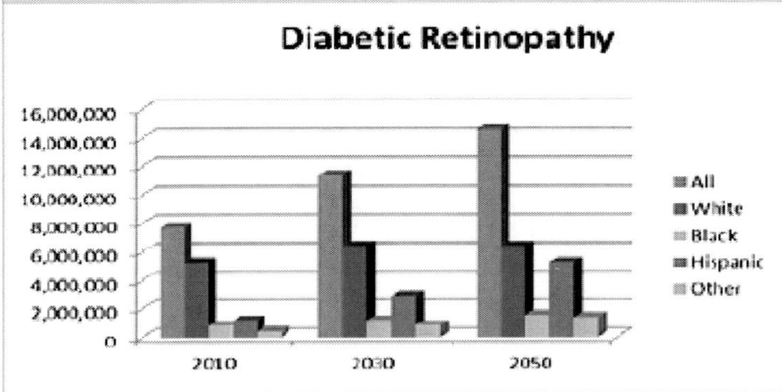


*Source: Vision Problems in the United States 2012*

Remember, if you have diabetes, make annual comprehensive dilated eye exams part of your self- management routine. Living with diabetes can be challenging, but you don't have to lose your vision or go blind because of it. To help friends and loved ones reduce their risk, please share this article.

For more information on diabetic eye disease, tips on finding an eye care professional, or information on financial assistance, visit https://www.nei.nih.gov/diabetes or call NEI at 301–496–5248.

NEI leads the federal government's research on the visual system and eye diseases. NEI supports basic and clinical science programs to develop sight-saving treatments and address special needs of people with vision loss. For more information, visit https://www.nei.nih.gov/

NIH, the Nation's medical research agency, includes 27 Institutes and Centers and is a component of the U.S. Department of Health and Human Services. NIH is the primary federal agency conducting and supporting basic, clinical, and translational medical research, and investigating the causes, treatments, and cures for both common and rare diseases. For more information about NIH and its programs, visit https://www.nih.gov.

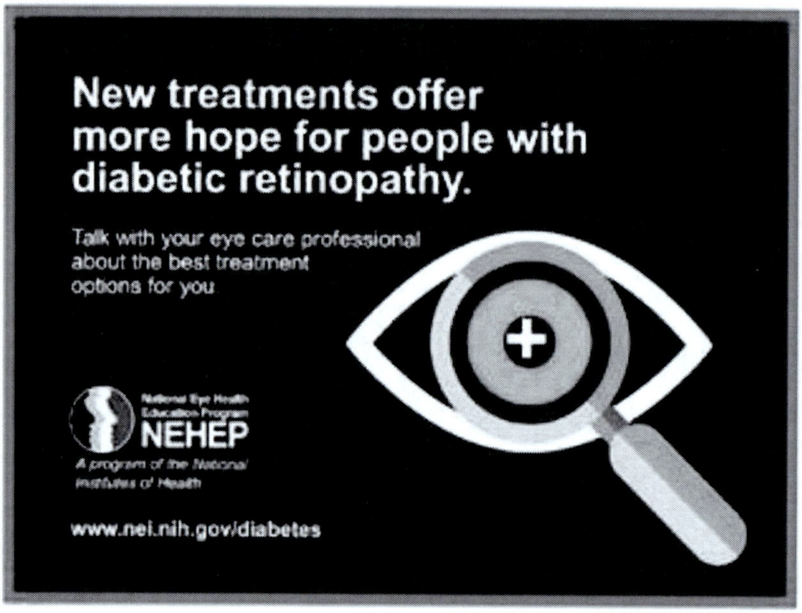


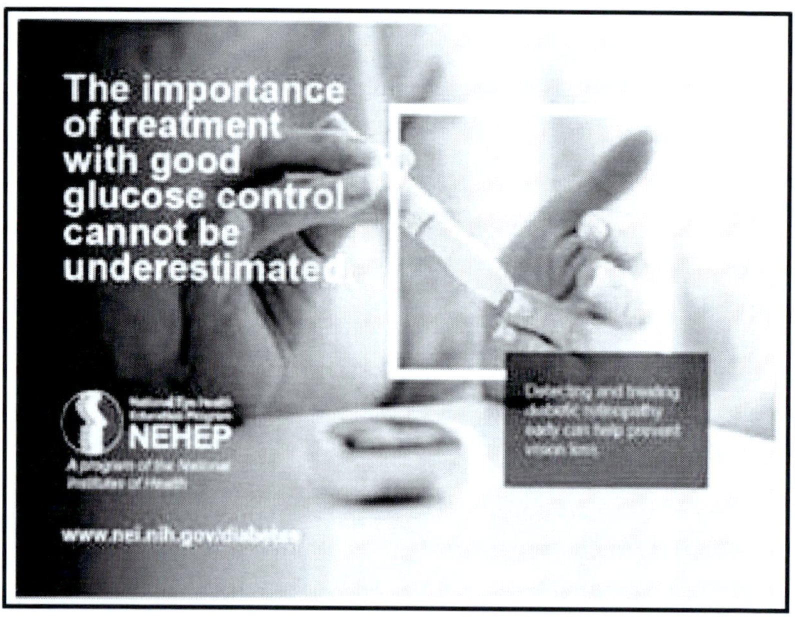

## Chapter 15

# Diabetic Eye Disease: Stay on TRACK to Prevent Blindness from Diabetes*


## National Eye Institute


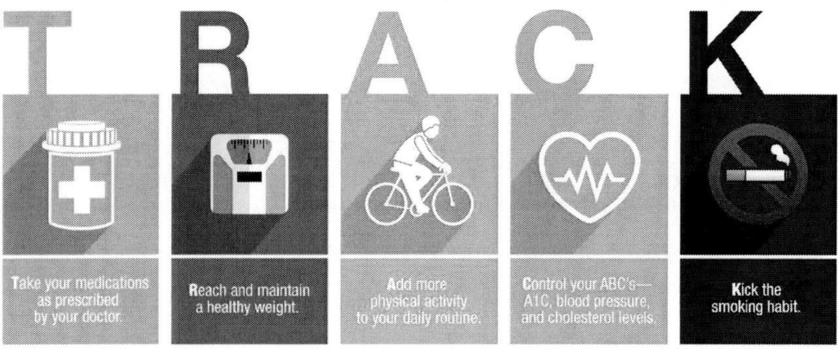


### Eleven Million People to Be at Risk by 2030

You can't feel it. You can't see it—until it's too late. Diabetic retinopathy, the most common form of diabetic eye disease, is the leading cause of blindness in adults age 20–74. It occurs when diabetes damages blood vessels in the retina.

Diabetic retinopathy affects 7.7 million Americans, and that number is projected to increase to more than 11 million people by 2030.

* This is an edited, reformatted and augmented version of the National Institutes of Health, National Eye Institute Publication.


In: Comprehensive Diabetes Care
Editor: Joseph S. Green
ISBN: 979-8-89530-772-4

Dr. Paul Sieving, director of the National Eye Institute (NEI), says, "Only about half of all people with diabetes get an annual comprehensive dilated eye exam, which is essential for detecting diabetic eye disease early, when it is most treatable."

With no early symptoms, diabetic eye disease—a group of conditions including cataract, glaucoma, and diabetic retinopathy—can affect anyone with type 1 or type 2 diabetes. African Americans, American Indians/Alaska Natives, and Hispanics/Latinos are at higher risk for losing vision or going blind from diabetes. The longer a person has diabetes, the greater the risk for diabetic eye disease. Once vision is lost, it often cannot be restored.

Keeping diabetes under control is key to slowing the progression of vision complications like diabetic retinopathy. There are important steps people with diabetes can take to keep their health on TRACK:

- Take your medications as prescribed by your doctor.
- Reach and maintain a healthy weight.
- Add physical activity to your daily routine.
- Control your ABC's—A1C, blood pressure, and cholesterol levels.
- Kick the smoking habit.

Additionally, people with diabetes should have annual comprehensive dilated eye exams to help protect their sight. Early detection, timely treatment, and appropriate follow-up care can reduce a person's risk for severe vision loss from diabetic eye disease by 95 percent.

"More than ever, it's important for people with diabetes to have a comprehensive dilated eye exam at least once a year. New treatments are being developed all the time, and we are learning that different treatments may work best for different patients. What hasn't changed is that early treatment is always better," says Dr. Suber Huang, chair of the Diabetic Eye Disease Subcommittee for NEI's National Eye Health Education Program (NEHEP) and member of the NEI-funded Diabetic Retinopathy Clinical Research Network (DRCR.net). "There has never been a more hopeful time in the treatment of diabetic retinopathy," he adds.

## Did You Know?

- Diabetes affects more than 9 percent of the U.S. population.

- More than 1 in 3 people have prediabetes.
- Everyone with diabetes is at risk for diabetic retinopathy—the number one cause of vision loss and blindness in working-age adults.

## Projected Increase of Diabetic Retinopathy in the United States, by Ethnicity

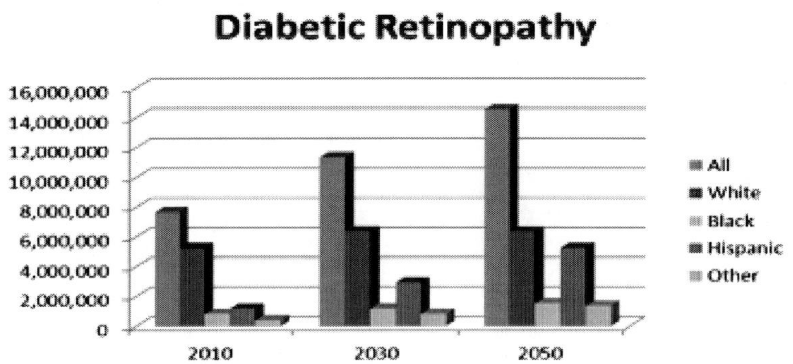


*Source: Vision Problems in the United States, 2012*

Remember, if you have diabetes, make annual comprehensive dilated eye exams part of your self- management routine. Living with diabetes can be challenging, but you don't have to lose your vision or go blind because of it. To help friends and loved ones reduce their risk, share this article.

For more information on diabetic eye disease, tips on finding an eye care professional, or information on financial assistance, visit http://www.nei.nih.gov/diabetes or call NEI at 301–496–5248.

The National Eye Institute (NEI), part of the National Institutes of Health (NIH), leads the federal government's research on the visual system and eye diseases. NEI supports basic and clinical science programs that result in the development of sight-saving treatments. For more information, visit http://www.nei.nih.gov.

NIH, the Nation's medical research agency, includes 27 Institutes and Centers and is a component of the U.S. Department of Health and Human Services. NIH is the primary federal agency conducting and supporting basic, clinical, and translational medical research, and investigating the causes, treatments, and cures for both common and rare diseases. For more information about NIH and its programs, visit http://www.nih.gov.

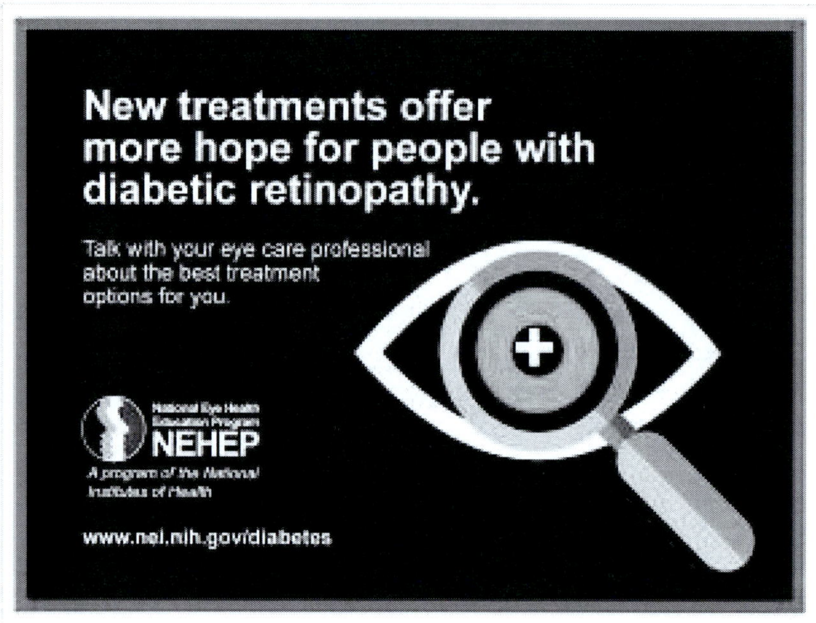


To learn more, visit http://www.nei.nih.gov/diabetes.

# Chapter 16

# Intermittent Fasting and Type 2 Diabetes*

## National Institutes of Health

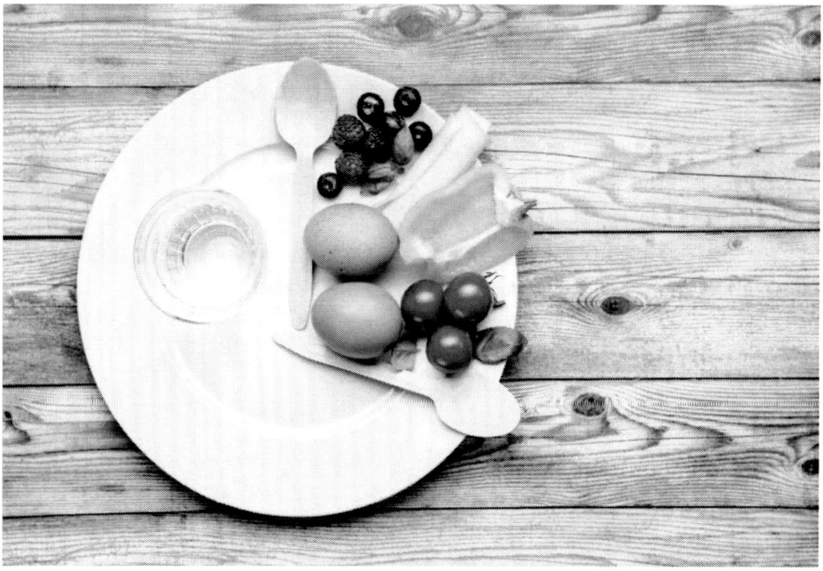

Around 1 in 10 Americans live with type 2 diabetes. In this disease, levels of blood glucose, or blood sugar, stay too high for too long. Diabetes can lead to serious health issues.

Weight loss is often recommended for those with excess weight and type 2 diabetes. Reducing calorie intake is a common weight-loss strategy. But many people find it hard to cut back on calories.

---

* This is an edited, reformatted and augmented version of National Institutes of Health Publication.

In: Comprehensive Diabetes Care
Editor: Joseph S. Green
ISBN: 979-8-89530-772-4

An NIH-funded research team tested a different strategy. It's called time-restricted eating, or intermittent fasting. With this approach, people eat only during a certain time period each day. During that time, they can eat anything they want.

The researchers recruited 75 people with obesity and type 2 diabetes. Participants were assigned to one of three diet groups. One group tried intermittent fasting. They ate only between noon and 8 p.m. Another group was asked to reduce their calorie intake by 25%. A third group had no dietary changes.

After six months, people in the fasting group had lost an average of 3.6% of their body weight. In comparison, people in the reduced-calorie group did not lose much weight. Both groups had similarly healthy decreases in blood glucose levels.

"Our study shows that time-restricted eating might be an effective alternative to traditional dieting for people who can't do the traditional diet or are burned out on it," says Dr. Krista Varady of the University of Illinois Chicago. For safety, people with diabetes who want to try intermittent fasting should talk to their doctor first.

# Chapter 17

# Diabetes Tests and Diagnosis*


## National Institute of Diabetes and Digestive and Kidney Diseases


Your doctor can diagnose diabetes, prediabetes, and gestational diabetes using blood tests. The blood tests show if your blood glucose level, also called blood sugar, is higher than the range that is healthy for you. Blood tests can also help identify the type of diabetes you have.

Don't try to diagnose yourself if you think you might have diabetes. Blood testing equipment that you can buy over the counter, such as a blood glucose meter, cannot diagnose diabetes.

## Who Should Be Tested for Diabetes?

Anyone who has symptoms of diabetes should be tested for the disease. Some people will not have any symptoms but may have risk factors for type 2 diabetes and need to be tested. Most pregnant women should also be tested for gestational diabetes. Testing helps doctors find diabetes sooner, so they can work with their patients to manage the disease and prevent health problems.

If you have Medicare, it may cover the cost of tests if you have certain risk factors External link for diabetes. If you have different insurance, ask your insurance company if it covers diabetes tests.

---

* This is an edited, reformatted and augmented version of National Institute of Diabetes and Digestive and Kidney Diseases Publication.


In: Comprehensive Diabetes Care
Editor: Joseph S. Green
ISBN: 979-8-89530-772-4

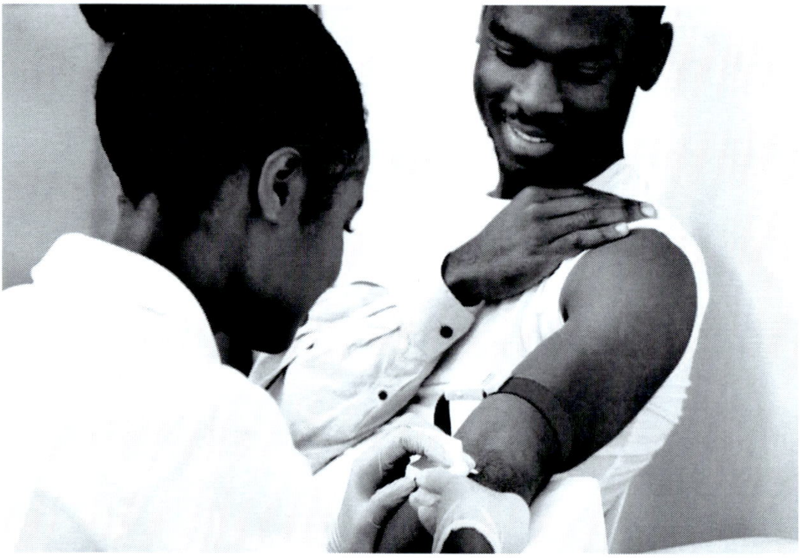

Blood tests help doctors diagnose diabetes and prediabetes.

## Type 1 Diabetes

Doctors often diagnose type 1 diabetes in children and young adults when they have diabetes symptoms, such as feeling thirsty and having to urinate more often, or if they may have diabetic ketoacidosis External link. Symptoms in adults may be less specific [1].

Type 1 diabetes can run in families. A study called TrialNet External link offers free testing to relatives of people with type 1 diabetes, even if the relatives don't have symptoms.

## Type 2 Diabetes

Experts recommend routine testing for type 2 diabetes if you have certain risk factors. You may have a higher risk of developing type 2 diabetes if you are

- age 35 or older
- American Indian, Black or African American, Asian American, Hispanic/Latino, or Pacific Islander

- overweight or have obesity and have at least one other risk factor
- a woman who had gestational diabetes

Take the American Diabetes Association Diabetes Risk Test to see if you are at risk for type 2 diabetes.

Children can also develop type 2 diabetes. Experts recommend testing children and teens between the ages of 10 and 18 who are overweight or have obesity and have at least one more risk factor, such as a low birth weight, a parent who had diabetes while pregnant, or another factor.1

Adults and children with normal diabetes test results should be retested every 3 years [1].

If your blood glucose levels are higher than the target range, but not high enough to be diagnosed with diabetes, doctors will diagnose you with prediabetes. Having prediabetes is serious because it raises the chance of developing type 2 diabetes. But developing type 2 diabetes can be prevented. Adults and children diagnosed with prediabetes should be tested for type 2 diabetes every year.

## Testing for Type 2 Diabetes Before and During Pregnancy

All women who are planning to get pregnant should be tested for type 2 diabetes, especially if they have risk factors.

If you are already pregnant, you should be tested for type 2 diabetes at the first prenatal appointment, or in the first 15 weeks of pregnancy. If you have diabetes, you should receive special care during your pregnancy to avoid problems for you and the baby.

## Gestational Diabetes

All pregnant women who do not have a previous diagnosis of diabetes should be tested for gestational diabetes between 24 and 28 weeks of pregnancy [1].

If you have gestational diabetes, you should get tested after your baby is born to see if you have type 2 diabetes, usually within 12 weeks after delivery.

## What Tests Are Used to Diagnose Diabetes?

Doctors use a variety of tests to diagnose diabetes and prediabetes. Your doctor may recommend different tests depending on whether you have symptoms or not, or whether you are pregnant.

### Fasting Plasma Glucose Test

The fasting plasma glucose (FPG) test measures your blood glucose level at a single point in time. For the most reliable results, your doctor will give you the test in the morning after you have fasted for at least 8 hours. Fasting means having nothing to eat or drink except sips of water.

### A1C Test

The A1C test is a blood test that provides your average levels of blood glucose over the last 3 months. Other names for the A1C test are hemoglobin A1C, HbA1C, glycated hemoglobin, and glycosylated hemoglobin test. You can eat and drink before this test. Before using the A1C test to diagnose diabetes, your doctor will consider factors, such as whether you are in your second or third trimester of pregnancy or whether you have certain types of anemia *NIH external link* or another problem with your blood.[1] The A1C test might not be accurate in those cases.

Certain types of hemoglobin, called hemoglobin variants, can interfere with measuring A1C levels. Most A1C tests used in the United States are not affected by the most common variants. If your A1C test results and blood glucose levels do not match, your doctor should consider that the A1C test may not be a reliable test for you.

Your doctor will report your A1C test result as a percentage, such as an A1C of 7%. The higher the percentage is, the higher your average blood glucose levels are.

## Random Plasma Glucose Test

Sometimes doctors use the random plasma glucose test to diagnose diabetes when you have symptoms of diabetes and they do not want to wait until you have fasted for 8 hours. You may have this blood test at any time.

## Glucose Challenge Test

If you are pregnant, your doctor might test you for gestational diabetes with the glucose challenge test. Another name for this test is the glucose screening test. In this test, a health care professional will take a sample of your blood 1 hour after you drink a sweet liquid containing glucose. You do not need to fast for this test. If your blood glucose level is too high—135 mg/dL to 140 mg/dL or higher—you may need to return for an oral glucose tolerance test while fasting.

## Oral Glucose Tolerance Test

The oral glucose tolerance test (OGTT) helps doctors detect type 2 diabetes, prediabetes, and gestational diabetes. However, the OGTT is a more expensive test than the FPG test and the glucose challenge test, and it is not as easy to give.

Before the test, you will need to fast for at least 8 hours. A health care professional will take a blood sample to measure your glucose level after fasting. Next, you will drink a liquid that is high in sugar. Another blood sample is taken 2 hours later to check your blood glucose level. If your blood glucose level is high, you may have diabetes.

If you are pregnant, your blood will be drawn every hour for 2 to 3 hours. If your blood glucose levels are high two or more times during the OGTT, you may have gestational diabetes.

## What Test Results Tell Me If I Have Diabetes or Prediabetes?

Each test to detect diabetes and prediabetes uses a different measurement. Usually, your doctor will use a second test to confirm you have diabetes.

The table below helps you understand what your test results mean if you are not pregnant [1]. If you are pregnant, some tests use different cutoffs. Ask your doctor what your test results mean.

## Test Results for Diagnosis of Prediabetes and Diabetes

| Diagnosis | A1C | Fasting Plasma Glucose | Oral Glucose Tolerance Test* | Random Plasma Glucose Test‡ |
|---|---|---|---|---|
| Normal | below 5.7% | 99 mg/dL or below | 139 mg/dL or below | N/A |
| Prediabetes | 5.7% to 6.4% | 100 to 125 mg/dL | 140 to 199 mg/dL | N/A |
| Diabetes | 6.5% or above | 126 mg/dL or above | 200 mg/dL or above | 200 mg/dL or above |

Source: American Diabetes Association.
* 2 hours after glucose intake
‡ Used when there are symptoms

## Which Tests Help My Doctor Know What Kind of Diabetes I Have?

Even though the tests described above can confirm you have diabetes, they can't identify what type you have—type 1, type 2, or a rare type of diabetes called monogenic diabetes. Treatment can depend on the type of diabetes you have, so knowing which type you have is important.

## Genetic Testing

Genetic testing can diagnose most forms of monogenic diabetes, which is caused by a change—or mutation—in a gene. Anyone can have monogenic diabetes, but it is more common in babies who develop diabetes before they are 6 months old, some teens, and some young adults.

## Autoantibodies

If you have diabetes, your doctor may look for certain autoantibodies to see if your diabetes is type 1. Autoantibodies are proteins in your immune system that mistakenly attack your healthy tissues and cells. A health care professional will take a sample of your blood for this test. If autoantibodies for diabetes are found in your blood, you may have type 1 diabetes [1].

If you do not have diabetes but your parent or sibling has type 1 diabetes, your doctor might give you this test to see if you have a higher risk of developing type 1 diabetes. You may want to learn about diabetes symptoms and have follow-up testing as recommended by your doctor [1].

## Reference

[1] American Diabetes Association Professional Practice Committee. Standards of medical care in diabetes—2022. *Diabetes Care*. 2022;45(suppl 1):1–16.7.

# Chapter 18

# Diabetes Medicines*

## U.S. Food and Drug Administration

Diabetes can make it hard to control how much sugar (called glucose) is in your blood.

### There Is Hope!

Some people with diabetes can take medicines to help keep their blood sugar at a healthy level.

This booklet gives some basic facts about diabetes medicines. Insulin is covered in a separate booklet.

People with type 1 diabetes must use insulin.

Use this booklet to help you talk to your healthcare provider about the kind of medicine that is right for you.

### Do Not Wait. Diabetes Is a Serious Illness

Diabetes can cause a heart attack, stroke, blindness, kidney disease, nerve damage, and other serious health problems. This is why it is so important for you to get treatment for your diabetes. Treatment can help prevent or slow some of these serious health problems.

---

* This is an edited, reformatted and augmented version of U.S. Food and Drug Administration Publication, dated 2018.

In: Comprehensive Diabetes Care
Editor: Joseph S. Green
ISBN: 979-8-89530-772-4

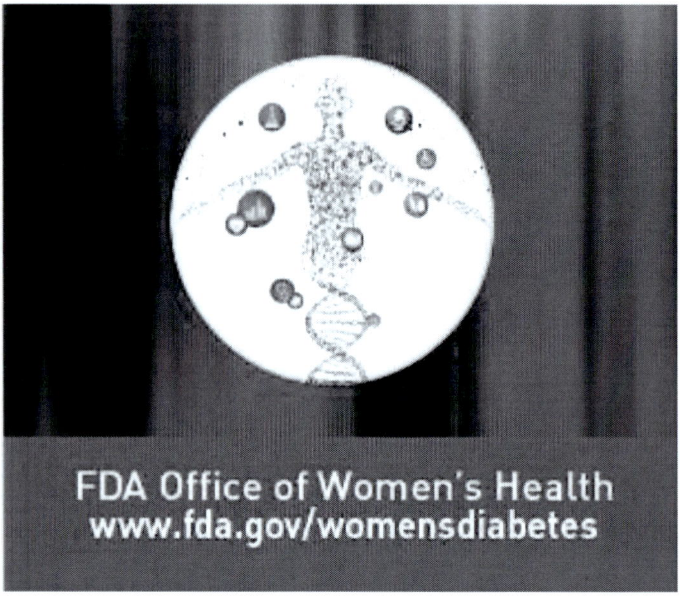


## You Can Control Your Diabetes

### Diabetes Tips

Talk to your healthcare provider before you change or stop taking your diabetes medicines.

Ask your healthcare provider about:

- your target blood sugar level.
- what you should do if your blood sugar gets too low or too high.
- how your diabetes medicines will affect your other medicines including birth control.

There are a few kinds of medicines used to treat diabetes. Each kind affects your body in a different way. Some diabetes medicines are taken as pills that you swallow. There are other medicines that you inject.

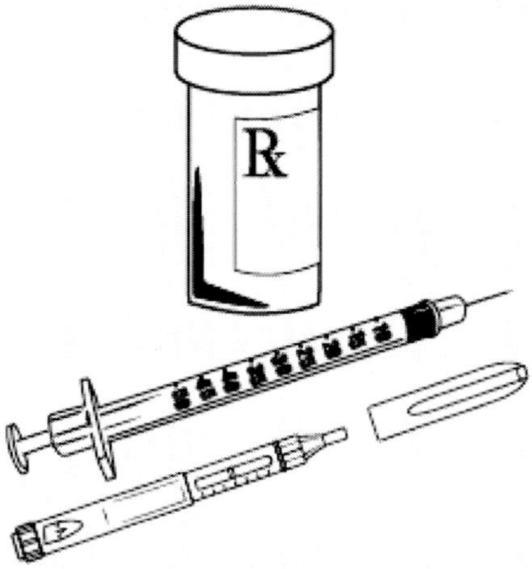


Some people with diabetes need to use medicines every day. What you need depends on your health and the type of diabetes you have. Your healthcare provider can tell you if you need to use medicine to treat your diabetes.

## Do I Need To Take Diabetes Medicines?

Some people with diabetes need to use medicines every day. What you need depends on your health and the type of diabetes you have. *Your healthcare provider can tell you if you need to use medicine to treat your diabetes.*

| | |
|---|---|
| Type 1 Diabetes | People with type 1 diabetes make very little or no insulin in their bodies. They must take insulin every day to stay alive. |
| Type 2 Diabetes | People with type 2 diabetes do not make enough insulin or do not use it well enough. Some people with type 2 diabetes can use pills or take other medicines as shots. Other people with type 2 diabetes need insulin to help control their diabetes. |
| Gestational Diabetes | Some women get diabetes for the first time when they become pregnant. This is called gestational (jes-TAY-shun-ul) diabetes.<br>Some women with gestational diabetes need to use insulin to control their blood sugar. |

## What You Can Do About Side Effects

Diabetes medicines do not act the same in each person. These medicines can sometimes cause side effects. The side effects will depend on your body and the type of medicine you are taking. Follow these tips to help you learn how to handle the side effects.

- Get the facts. Ask your healthcare provider for the side effects, warnings, and other facts for the medicines you are taking. This booklet does not give all facts for each kind of diabetes medicine.
- Speak up. Tell someone about any problems you may be having with your medicines. Your doctor may change your medicine or give you tips to help you deal with the side effects.
- Check the FDA website. You can find current safety information about your medicine at: www.fda.gov
- Report serious problems with your medicines. You or your doctor can tell the FDA about serious problems with your medicines.

*Report Online at: www.fda.gov/medwatch*
*Call 1-800-FDA-1088 to request a form.*

## Diabetes Tip

Talk to your doctor *before* you change or stop taking your diabetes medicines.

Different kinds of diabetes medicines are shown on the next few pages. These medicines are most often used to treat type 2 diabetes. The brand names and other names are given for each medicine. There are also some tips about each kind of diabetes medicine. Ask your healthcare provider to tell you the best way to take your medicines. They can also tell you about your medicine's side effects and warnings. *This guide does not give all side effects or warnings for each medicine.*

## Meglitinides

How do they work? These pills help your body make more insulin around mealtime.

| BRAND NAME | OTHER NAME |
|---|---|
| Prandin | repaglinide |
| Starlix | nateglinide |

## Some Things to Think About

Before you start taking these medicines, tell your healthcare provider if:

- you have liver or kidney problems.
- you are pregnant or breastfeeding.

## Common Side Effects

Hypoglycemia (blood sugar that is too low)

## Alpha-Glucosidase Inhibitors

*How do they work?* These pills help your body digest sugar more slowly.

| BRAND NAME | OTHER NAME |
|---|---|
| Glyset | miglitol |
| Precose | acarbose |

## Some Things to Think About

Before you start taking these medicines, tell your healthcare provider if:

- you have heart, liver, or kidney problems.
- you are pregnant or breastfeeding.

These medicines are not likely to cause low blood sugar or weight gain.

## Common Side Effects

- Stomach Pain
- Diarrhea
- Gas
- Abnormal Liver Tests

## Thiazolidinediones

How do they work? These pills help the cells in your body use glucose.

| BRAND NAME | OTHER NAME |
|---|---|
| Actos | pioglitazone |
| Avandia | rosiglitazone |

## Some Things to Think About

- Before you start taking these medicines, tell your doctor if you have heart problems or heart failure.
- These medicines may raise your chance of having a broken bone (fracture).
- Before you take Actos, tell your doctor if you are a premenopausal woman (before the "change of life") who does not have periods regularly or at all. Actos may increase your chance of becoming pregnant. Talk to your doctor about birth control choices while taking Actos.

## Common Side Effects

- Fluid Retention
- Weight Gain
- Heart Failure (heart cannot pump blood well)

- Anemia (low red blood cell counts)
- Upper Respiratory Tract Infection

## DPP- 4 Inhibitors

*How do they work?* These pills help your body release more insulin.

| BRAND NAME | OTHER NAME |
|---|---|
| Januvia | sitagliptin |
| Onglyza | saxagliptin |
| Nesina | alogliptin |
| Tradjenta | linagliptin |

## Some Things to Think About

- Call your doctor right away if you have severe stomach pain or vomiting. This may be a sign of a serious side effect.

## Common Side Effects

- Upper Respiratory Infection
- Headache

## Sulfonylureas

*How do they work?* These pills help your body make more insulin.

| BRAND NAME | OTHER NAME |
|---|---|
| Amaryl | glimepiride |
| Diabeta<br>Glynase | glyburide |
| Diabinese | chlorpropamide |
| Glucotrol Glucotrol XL<br>(Extended release) | glipizide |
| No brand name | tolbutamide |
| No brand name | tolazamide |

## Some Things to Think About

- Before you start taking these drugs, tell your doctor if you have heart, liver, or kidney problems.
- Older adults and people with kidney or liver problems may be more likely to have low blood sugar when taking these medicines.

## Common Side Effects

- Hypoglycemia
- Weight Gain (blood sugar that is too low)
- Headache
- Dizziness

## Biguanides

How do they work? These pills stop your liver from making too much sugar (glucose). They also help the sugar get into your cells.

| BRAND NAME | OTHER NAME |
|---|---|
| Fortamet | metformin |
| Glucophage | metformin |
| Glucophage XR (long-lasting extended release) | metformin |
| Glumetza | metformin |
| Riomet | metformin |

## Some Things to Think About

- Talk to your doctor about your kidney health before you start and while you are taking this type of medicine.
- These medicines are not likely to cause low blood sugar or weight gain.

- People who drink a lot of alcohol and people with kidney problems may have a rare side effect called lactic acidosis (acid build up in the blood).

## Common Side Effects

- Diarrhea
- Indigestion
- Nausea/Vomiting
- Gas
- Feeling Weak
- Headache

## Dopamine Receptor Agonists

How do they work? This pill affects a chemical called dopamine in your cells. It is not clear how this pill works for diabetes.

| BRAND NAME | OTHER NAME |
|---|---|
| Cycloset | bromocriptine |

## Some Things to Think About

- Do not take this medicine if you are breastfeeding.

### Common Side Effects

- Nausea
- Headache
- Feel Very Tired
- Feel Dizzy
- Vomiting

## Bile Acid Sequestrants

How do they work? It is not clear how this pill works for diabetes.

| BRAND NAME | OTHER NAME |
|---|---|
| Welchol | colesevelam |

## Some Things to Think About

- This medicine is also used to treat high cholesterol.
- Tell your doctor if you are taking other cholesterol medicines.

## Common Side Effects

- Constipation
- Dyspepsia (upset stomach/indigestion)
- Nausea

## SGLT2 Inhibitors

How do they work? These pills affect the kidney to increase the amount of sugar that goes out in the urine.

| BRAND NAME | OTHER NAME |
|---|---|
| Farxiga | dapagliflozin |
| Invokana | canagliflozin |
| Jardiance | empagliflozin |
| Steglatro | ertugliflozin |

## Some Things to Think About

- Do not take these drugs if you have severe kidney problems or are on dialysis.

- Before you take these drugs, tell your doctor if you have kidney or Liver problems.

## Common Side Effects

- Vaginal Yeast Infections
- Urinary Tract Infections
- Changes in Urination

## Combination Medicines

These combinations are made up of two kinds of medicines. Ask your healthcare provider for the facts about the combination drug you are taking.

| BRAND NAME | OTHER NAME |
|---|---|
| ActoPlus Met<br>ActoPlus Met XR | pioglitazone and metformin |
| Avandamet | rosiglitazone and metformin |
| Avandaryl | rosiglitazone and glimepiride |
| Duetact | pioglitazone and glimepiride |
| Glucovance | glyburide and metformin |
| Glyxambi | empagliflozin and linagliptin |
| Invokamet<br>Invokamet XR | canagliflozin and metformin |
| Janumet<br>Janumet XR | sitagliptin and metformin |
| Jentadueto | linagliptin and metformin |
| Kazano | alogliptin and metformin |
| Kombiglyze<br>Kombiglyze XR | saxagliptin and metformin |
| Metaglip | glipizide and metformin |
| Oseni | alogliptin and pioglitazone |
| PrandiMet | repaglinide and metformin |
| Xigduo XR | dapagliflozin and metformin |

## GLP-1 Receptor Agonists

These are medicines that you inject under your skin. These medicines should not be used instead of insulin.

| BRAND NAME | OTHER NAME |
|---|---|
| Adlyxin | lixisenatide |
| Bydureon | exenatide |
| Byetta | exenatide |
| Ozempic | semaglutide |
| Tanzeum | albiglutide |
| Trulicity | dulaglutide |
| Victoza | liraglutide |

## Some Things to Think About

- These medicines are not the same as insulin.
- Some people feel nauseous when they first start taking these medicines.

## Amylin Analog

This is a medicine that you inject under your skin. This medicine should not be used instead of insulin.

| BRAND NAME | OTHER NAME |
|---|---|
| Symlin | pramlintide acetate |

## Some Things to Think About

- People who use insulin can also use Symlin.
- People with type 1 diabetes can use Symlin.
- Symlin should be taken in a separate injection. Do not mix Symlin and insulin in the same injection.
- This medicine is usually taken before meals.
- Some people feel nauseous when they first start taking this medicine.

| MEDICINE NAME | HOW MUCH DO I TAKE? | WHEN DO I TAKE IT? | IMPORTANT FACTS |
|---|---|---|---|
| | | | |
| | | | |
| | | | |
| | | | |

*Write down the facts about your diabetes medicines the next time you talk to your doctor, nurse, or diabetes educator.*

- How will my medicines affect my blood sugar?
- Will it affect my other medicines?
- What are the side effects?
- What do I do if I start having side effects?
- What should I do if I am pregnant, planning to get pregnant, or breastfeeding?
- What else should I know about my diabetes medicines?

______________________________________________

______________________________________________

______________________________________________

______________________________________________

______________________________________________

______________________________________________

______________________________________________

## Sign up for a Pregnancy Registry

Pregnancy Exposure Registries are research studies that collect information from women who take prescription medicines or vaccines during pregnancy.

Pregnancy registries can help women and their doctors learn more about how diabetes medicines affect women during pregnancy.

The FDA does not run pregnancy studies, but it keeps a list of registries.

Check to see if there is a registry for your diabetes medicine or other medicines at: www.fda.gov/pregnancyregistries

*This booklet should not be used in place of talking to your doctor or reading the label on your medicine. This booklet does not list all of the benefits or risks of taking these medicines. The drug and risk information in this booklet may change.*

*Check the FDA website for the latest facts on each medicine: www.accessdata.fda.gov/scripts/cder/drugsatfda/*

## You Can Control Your Diabetes

**Make a plan.**
Work with your doctor, nurse, or diabetes educator to plan how you will manage your diabetes.

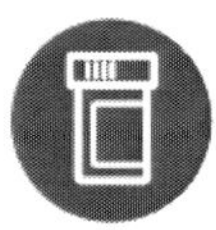

**Use medicines wisely.**
Ask your healthcare provider when and how to safely use your diabetes medicines or insulin.

**Check your blood sugar.**
Use your glucose meter to test your blood glucose (sugar) level during the day.

**Be active and get exercise.**
Dance, take a walk, or join an exercise class. Check with your healthcare provider about safe ways to be more active.

**Watch what you eat.**
Work with your healthcare team to make a meal plan just for you.

**Watch your overall mental and physical health.**
Work with your healthcare team to keep your feet, eyes, heart, and teeth healthy.

# Chapter 19

# Insulin, Medicines, and Other Diabetes Treatments*


## National Institute of Diabetes and Digestive and Kidney Diseases


Taking insulin or other diabetes medicines is often part of treating diabetes. In addition to making healthy food and beverage choices, getting physical activity, getting enough sleep, and managing stress, medicines can help you manage the disease. Some other treatment options are also available.

## What Medicines Might I Take for Diabetes?

The medicine you take depends on the type of diabetes you have and how well the medicine controls your blood glucose levels, also called blood sugar levels. Other factors, such as any other health conditions you may have, medication costs, your insurance coverage and copays, access to care, and your lifestyle, may affect what diabetes medicine you take.

* This is an edited, reformatted and augmented version of National Institute of Diabetes and Digestive and Kidney Diseases Publication.


In: Comprehensive Diabetes Care
Editor: Joseph S. Green
ISBN: 979-8-89530-772-4

## What Type of Diabetes Do I Have?

### Type 1 Diabetes

If you have type 1 diabetes, you must take insulin because your pancreas does not make it. You will need to take insulin several times during the day, including when you eat and drink, to control your blood glucose level.

There are different ways to take insulin. You can use a needle and syringe, an insulin pen, or an insulin pump. An artificial pancreas—also called an automated insulin delivery system—may be another option for some people.

### Type 2 Diabetes

Some people with type 2 diabetes can control their blood glucose level by making lifestyle changes. These lifestyle changes include consuming healthy meals and beverages, limiting calories if they have overweight or obesity, and getting physical activity.

Many people with type 2 diabetes need to take diabetes medicines as well. These medicines may include diabetes pills or medicines you inject, such as insulin. Over time, you may need more than one diabetes medicine to control your blood glucose level. Even if you do not take insulin, you may need it at special times, such as if you are pregnant or if you are in the hospital for treatment.

### Gestational Diabetes

If you have gestational diabetes, you can manage your blood glucose level by following a healthy eating plan and doing a moderate-intensity physical activity, such as brisk walking for 150 minutes, each week. If consuming healthy food and beverages and getting regular physical activity aren't enough to keep your blood glucose level in your target range, a doctor will work with you and may recommend you take insulin. Insulin is safe to take while you are pregnant.

No matter what type of diabetes you have, taking diabetes medicines every day can feel like a burden sometimes. New medications and improved delivery systems can help make it easier to manage your blood glucose levels.

Talk with your doctor to find out which medications and delivery systems will work best for you and fit into your lifestyle.

## What Are the Different Types of Insulin?

Several types of insulin are available. Each type starts to work at a different speed, known as "onset," and its effects last a different length of time, known as "duration." Most types of insulin reach a peak, which is when they have the strongest effect. After the peak, the effects of the insulin wear off over the next few hours or so. Table 1 lists the different types of insulin, how fast they start to work, when they peak, and how long they last.

**Table 1.** Types of insulin and how they work [1, 2]

| Insulin Type | How Fast It Starts to Work (onset) | When It Peaks | How Long It Lasts (duration) |
|---|---|---|---|
| rapid-acting/ ultra rapid-acting | 15 minutes | 1 hour | 2 to 4 hours (rapid) 5 to 7 hours (ultra) |
| rapid-acting, inhaled | 10 to 15 minutes | 30 minutes | 3 hours |
| regular, also called short-acting | 30 minutes | 2 to 3 hours | 3 to 6 hours |
| intermediate-acting | 2 to 4 hours | 4 to 12 hours | 12 to 18 hours |
| long-acting | 2 hours | does not peak | 24 hours |
| ultra long-acting | 6 hours | does not peak | 36 hours or longer |

Another type of insulin, called premixed insulin, is a combination of insulins listed in Table 1. Premixed insulin starts to work in 15 to 60 minutes and can last from 10 to 16 hours. The peak time varies depending on which insulins are mixed.

Your doctor will work with you to review your medication options. Talk with your doctor about your activity level, what you eat and drink, how well you manage your blood glucose levels, your age and lifestyle, and how long your body takes to absorb insulin.

Follow your doctor's advice on when and how to take your insulin. If you're worried about the cost, talk with your doctor. Some types of insulin cost more than others. You can also find resources to get financial help for diabetes care.

## What Are the Different Ways to Take Insulin?

The way you take insulin may depend on your lifestyle, insurance plan, and preferences. Talk with your doctor about the options and which one is best for you. Most people with diabetes take insulin using a needle and syringe, insulin pen, or insulin pump. Inhalers and insulin jet injectors are less common ways to take insulin. Artificial pancreas systems are now approved by the U.S. Food and Drug Administration (FDA). Talk with your doctor to see if an artificial pancreas is an option for you.

## Needle and Syringe

You can give yourself insulin shots using a needle and syringe. You draw up your dose of insulin from the vial—or bottle—through the needle into the syringe. Insulin works fastest when you inject it in your belly, but your doctor may recommend alternating the spot where you inject it. Injecting insulin in the same spot repeatedly could cause the tissue to harden, making it harder to take shots in that area over time. Other spots you can inject insulin include your thigh, buttocks, or upper arm, but it may take longer for the insulin to work from those areas. Some people with diabetes who take insulin need 2 to 4 shots a day to reach their blood glucose targets. Others can take a single shot. Injection aids can help you give yourself the shots.

### Pen

An insulin pen looks like a writing pen but has a needle for its point. Some insulin pens come filled with insulin and are disposable. Others have room for an insulin cartridge that you insert and replace after use. Many people find insulin pens easier to use, but they cost more than needles and syringes. You may want to consider using an insulin pen if you find it hard to fill the syringe while holding the vial or cannot read the markings on the syringe. Different pen types have features that can help with your injections. Some reusable pens have a memory function, which can recall dose amounts and timing. Other types of "connected" insulin pens can be programmed to calculate insulin doses and provide downloadable data reports, which can help you and your doctor adjust your insulin doses.

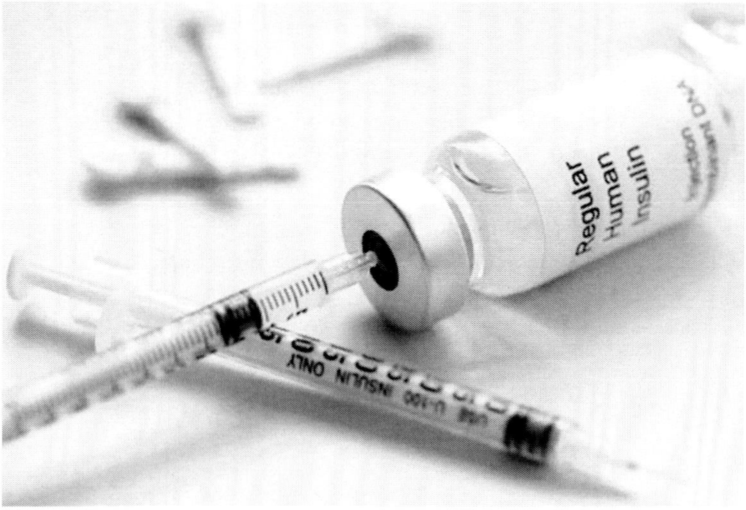


Insulin shots involve drawing insulin from a vial into a syringe and then injecting it.

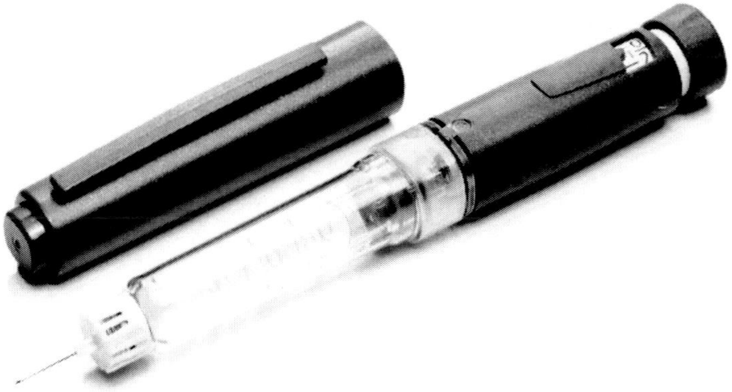

An insulin pen is a convenient way to take insulin.

### Pump

An insulin pump is a small machine that gives you steady doses of insulin throughout the day. You wear one type of pump outside your body on a belt or in a pocket or pouch. The insulin pump connects to a small plastic tube and a very small needle. You insert the plastic tube with a needle under your skin, then take out the needle. The plastic tube will stay inserted for several days while attached to the insulin pump. The machine pumps insulin through the tube into your body 24 hours a day and can be programmed to give you more or less insulin based on your needs. You can also give yourself doses of insulin through the pump at mealtimes.

Another type of pump has no tubes. This pump attaches directly to your skin with a self-adhesive pad and is controlled by a hand-held device. The plastic tube and pump device are changed every several days.

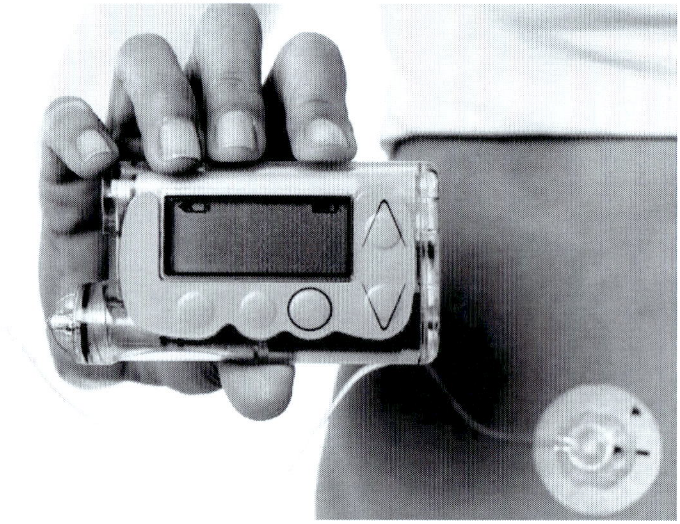

Insulin pumps can be programmed to deliver insulin directly into your body, 24 hours a day or at certain times.

### Inhaler

Another way to take insulin is by breathing powdered insulin into your mouth from an inhaler device. The insulin goes into your lungs and moves quickly into your blood. You may want to use an insulin inhaler *NIH external link* to avoid using needles. Inhaled insulin is only for adults with type 1 or type 2 diabetes. Taking insulin with an inhaler is less common than using a needle and syringe.

### Jet Injector

A jet injector is a device that sends a fine spray of insulin into the skin at high pressure instead of using a needle to deliver the insulin. It is used less commonly than a needle and syringe or a pen.

## Artificial Pancreas

An artificial pancreas is a system of three devices that work together to mimic how a healthy pancreas controls blood glucose in the body. A continuous glucose monitor (CGM) tracks blood glucose levels every few minutes using a small sensor inserted under the skin that is held in place with an adhesive pad. The CGM wirelessly sends the information to a program on a smartphone or an insulin infusion pump. The program calculates how much insulin you need. The insulin infusion pump will adjust how much insulin is given from minute to minute to help keep your blood glucose level in your target range. An artificial pancreas is mainly used to help people with type 1 diabetes.

## What Oral Medicines Treat Type 2 Diabetes?

You may need to take medicines to manage your type 2 diabetes, in addition to consuming healthy foods and beverages and being physically active. You can take many diabetes medicines by mouth. These medicines are called oral medicines.

Most people with type 2 diabetes start with metformin NIH external link pills. Metformin also comes as a liquid. Metformin helps your liver make less glucose and helps your body use insulin better. This drug may help you lose a small amount of weight.

Other oral medicines act in different ways to lower blood glucose levels. Combining two or three kinds of diabetes medicines can lower blood glucose levels better than taking just one medicine.

Read about different kinds of diabetes medicines External link (PDF, 2.8 MB) from the FDA.

## What Other Injectable Medicines Treat Diabetes?

### Type 1 Diabetes

If you have type 1 diabetes, your doctor may recommend you take other medicines, in addition to insulin, to help control your blood glucose. Some of these medicines work to slow how fast food and beverages move through your stomach. These medicines also slow down how quickly and how high your blood glucose levels rise after eating. Other medicines work to block certain hormones in your digestive system that raise blood glucose levels after meals or help the kidneys to remove more glucose from your blood.

### Type 2 Diabetes

Besides insulin, other types of injected medicines External link (PDF, 2.8 MB) are available that will keep your blood glucose level from rising too high after you eat or drink. These medicines, known as glucagon-like peptide-1 (GLP-1) receptor agonists, [3] may make you feel less hungry and help you lose some weight. GLP-1 medicines are not substitutes for insulin.

## What Should I Know About Side Effects of Diabetes Medicines?

Side effects are problems that result from taking a medicine. Some diabetes medicines can cause hypoglycemia, also called low blood glucose, if you don't balance your medicines with food and activity.

Ask your doctor whether your diabetes medicine can cause hypoglycemia or other side effects, such as upset stomach and weight gain. Aim to take your diabetes medicines as your doctor instructs you, to help prevent side effects and diabetes problems.

## What Questions Should I Ask About My Diabetes Medicines?

Ask your doctor these questions when you get a prescription for a medicine. You may want to make copies of this list and fill it out for each of your medicines.

1. What are the names of my medicine?

Brand name:______

Generic name:_____

2. What does my medicine do?
3. When should I start this medicine?
4. This medicine is prescribed by:_____
5. How long will this medicine take to work?
6. What is the strength (for example, how many milligrams, written as mg)?
7. How much should I take for each dose?
8. How many times a day should I take my medicine?
9. At what times should I take my medicine?
10. Should I take it before, with, or after a meal?
11. Should I avoid any foods or medicines when I take it?
12. Should I avoid alcoholic beverages when I take it?
13. Are there any times when I should change the amount of medicine I take?
14. What should I do if I forget to take it?
15. If I'm sick and can't keep food down, should I still take my medicine?
16. Can my diabetes medicine cause low blood glucose?
17. What should I do if my blood glucose is too low?
18. What side effects can this medicine cause?
19. What should I do if I have side effects?
20. How should I store this medicine?

## Do I Have Other Treatment Options for My Diabetes?

If medicines and lifestyle changes are not enough to manage your diabetes, there are other treatments that might help you. These treatments include weight-loss (bariatric) surgery for certain people with type 1 or type 2 diabetes, or pancreatic islet transplantation for some people with type 1 diabetes.

### Weight-Loss Surgery

Weight-loss surgery are operations that help you lose weight by making changes to your digestive system. Weight-loss surgery is also called bariatric or metabolic surgery.

This type of surgery may help some people who have obesity and type 2 diabetes lose a large amount of weight and bring their blood glucose levels back to a healthy range. How long the improved response lasts can vary by patient, type of weight-loss surgery, and the amount of weight the person lost. Other factors include how long a person had diabetes and whether the person used insulin. Some people with type 2 diabetes may no longer need to use diabetes medicines after weight-loss surgery [4].

Researchers are studying whether weight-loss surgery can help control blood glucose levels in people with type 1 diabetes who have obesity [5].

### Pancreatic Islet Transplantation

Pancreatic islet transplantation is a treatment for type 1 diabetes in people who struggle to manage their blood glucose levels. Pancreatic islets are clusters of cells in the pancreas that make the hormone insulin. In type 1 diabetes, the body's immune system attacks these cells. A pancreatic islet transplantation replaces destroyed islets with new islets from a deceased donor. The new islets make and release insulin.

## Clinical Trials For Insulin, Medicines, & Other Diabetes Treatments

The NIDDK conducts and supports clinical trials in many diseases and conditions, including diabetes. The trials look to find new ways to prevent, detect, or treat disease and improve quality of life.

## What are clinical trials for insulin, medicines, and other diabetes treatments?

- Clinical trials—and other types of clinical studies NIH external link—are part of medical research and involve people like you. When you volunteer to take part in a clinical study, you help health care professionals and researchers learn more about disease and improve health care for people in the future.
- Find out if clinical trials are right for you NIH external link.
- Researchers are studying many aspects of diabetes medicines, including
- new types of insulin
- the most effective times to take diabetes medicines
- new types of monitoring devices and delivery systems

Watch a video of NIDDK Director Dr. Griffin P. Rodgers explaining the importance of participating in clinical trials.

## What Clinical Trials for Insulin, Medicines, and Other Diabetes Treatments Are Looking for Participants?

You can view a filtered list of clinical studies on insulin, medicines, and other diabetes treatments covered in this health topic that are federally funded, open, and recruiting at www.ClinicalTrials.gov NIH external link. You can expand or narrow the list to include clinical studies from industry, universities, and individuals; however, the National Institutes of Health does not review these studies and cannot ensure they are safe. Always talk with your health care provider before you participate in a clinical study.

## References

[1] Types of insulin. Centers for Disease Control and Prevention. Updated March 25, 2021. Accessed January 24, 2022. www.cdc.gov/diabetes/basics/type-1-types-of-insulin.html External link.

[2] Wong EY, Kroon L. Ultra-rapid-acting insulins: how fast is really needed? *Clinical Diabetes*. 2021;39(4):415–423. doi:10.2337/cd20-0119.

[3] Collins L, Costello RA. Glucagon-like Peptide-1 Receptor Agonists. In: *StatPearls [Internet]*. StatPearls Publishing; 2021. Updated June 25, 2021. Accessed April 21, 2022. www.ncbi.nlm.nih.gov/books/NBK551568 *NIH external link.*

[4] Brethauer SA, Aminian A, Romero-Talamás H, et al. Can diabetes be surgically cured? Long-term metabolic effects of bariatric surgery in obese patients with type 2 diabetes mellitus *NIH external link*. *Annals of Surgery*. 2013;258(4):628–636. doi: 10.1097/SLA.0b013e3182a5034b.

[5] Vilarrasa N, San Jose P, Rubio MÁ, Lecube A. Obesity in patients with type 1 diabetes: links, risks, and management challenges. *Diabetes, Metabolic Syndrome, and Obesity: Targets and Therapy*. 2021;14:2807–2827. doi: 10.2147/DMSO.S223618.

## Chapter 20

# Medicare Coverage of GLP-1 Drugs*


## Laura A. Wreschnig


Glucagon-like peptide-1 (GLP-1) receptor agonists, marketed under brand names such as Wegovy and Ozempic, are a class of medications used primarily in the treatment of type 2 diabetes mellitus (T2DM). Recently, GLP-1 drugs have gained attention for their effectiveness in obesity treatment. Given the increasing prevalence of obesity amongst Medicare beneficiaries, the demand for GLP-1 drugs also has increased, leading to discussions about their coverage under Medicare's outpatient prescription drug benefit (Part D), the associated spending implications, and policy considerations for Congress. This In Focus provides a brief overview of GLP-1 drugs, their current coverage status under Medicare Part D, and related policy considerations.

### Overview of GLP-1 Drugs

Beginning in the 1980s, scientists realized that certain hormones played vital roles in the human body's regulation of insulin production. One of the key hormones is GLP-1, a gastrointestinal hormone released after eating. GLP-1 drugs mimic the effects of this hormone and therefore help regulate insulin production, which is a vital function for patients with T2DM.

The first GLP-1 drug, exenatide (brand name Byetta), was approved by the Food and Drug Administration (FDA) for the treatment of T2DM in 2005. As more GLP-1 drugs came on the market, researchers discovered additional benefits beyond managing T2DM. Clinical trials provided evidence that GLP-1 drugs were capable of slowing digestion, affecting areas of the brain that

* This is an edited, reformatted and augmented version of Congressional Research Service Publication No. IF12758, dated September 9, 2024.


In: Comprehensive Diabetes Care
Editor: Joseph S. Green
ISBN: 979-8-89530-772-4

process hunger, and thus reducing a patient's weight. In 2014, Saxendra (Liraglutide) was the first GLP-1 drug approved by the FDA for weight loss. In 2021, the FDA approved Novo Nordisk's application to market a GLP-1 drug for weight loss under the brand name Wegovy. In 2023, the FDA approved another GLP-1 drug for weight loss, tirzepatide, under the brand name Zepbound.

Not all GLP-1 drugs are FDA approved for weight loss. Despite its popularity as a weight loss treatment, Ozempic, another GLP-1 drug manufactured by Novo Nordisk, is only FDA approved for the treatment of T2DM. The delivery mechanism also differs within this class of drugs. Both Wegovy and Ozempic are injectable, but some GLP-1 drugs such as Rybelsus can be taken orally. There are indications that GLP-1 drugs could be used for conditions other than T2DM and weight loss. In March 2024, the FDA approved the use of Wegovy to reduce the risk of heart attack and stroke in adults with cardiovascular disease (CVD) who were either obese or overweight.

## Overview of Medicare Part D Benefit

Medicare Part D is a voluntary outpatient prescription drug benefit administered by private health payers (plan sponsors) through stand-alone Prescription Drug Plans (PDPs) or Medicare Advantage (MA) plans with a Part D benefit (MA-PD). Each year, the Centers for Medicare & Medicaid Services (CMS) issues guidance that defines a standard Part D benefit. The defined standard benefit sets limits on out-of-pocket (OOP) spending, deductibles, and cost sharing. CMS requires every Part D sponsor to offer at least one basic plan in a given service area that is either the standard benefit or actuarially equivalent to the standard benefit.

This basic coverage applies to all Part D-covered drugs. Part D-covered drugs are generally defined as FDA- approved drugs and vaccines that are on the formulary of a Part D plan and are not covered under Medicare Parts A or B. Part D plans must offer a formulary that covers substantially all drugs available in the six protected drug classes: immune-suppressant, antidepressant, antipsychotic, anticonvulsant, antiretroviral, and antineoplastic (cancer). Outside of the six protected classes, Part D drug plans are required to operate formularies that cover at least two drugs in each drug class and category but have flexibility over which drugs to offer.

## Coverage Under the Standard Benefit

Certain types of drugs are prohibited from being considered covered Part D drugs under the standard plan. The Medicare Prescription Drug, Improvement, and Modernization Act of 2003 (MMA; P.L. 108-173), which created Part D, excluded drugs used for anorexia, weight loss, or weight gain. The restrictions were based on the existing definition of drugs or classes of drugs that may be excluded from Medicaid coverage under Social Security Act Section 1927(d)(2). Therefore, GLP-1 drugs, even if they have received FDA approval for weight loss, are not covered under Part D drugs when used for that purpose.

Currently, Medicare allows coverage through Part D plans for GLP-1 drugs that the FDA has approved for T2DM and CVD. As of August 2024, Ozempic, Mounjaro, Rybelsus, and Wegovy are considered covered Part D drugs for the treatment of those conditions. Table 1 displays Medicare expenditures in 2022 for a subset of these covered GLP-1 drugs. Eligibility for Part D coverage does not ensure all Part D plans will include those GLP-1 drugs in their formulary. As described above, Part D plans are required to cover at least two drugs each for the treatment of T2DM and/or CVD, but it is not required that either drug be a GLP-1 drug.

**Table 1. 2022 medicare spend on selected GLP-1 drugs**

| Brand Name | Ozempic | Rybelsus | Mounjaro |
|---|---|---|---|
| Generic Name | Semaglutide | Semaglutide | Tirzepatide |
| Manufacturer | Novo Nordisk | Novo Nordisk | Eli Lilly & Co. |
| FDA Approval for | T2DM | T2DM | T2DM |
| Total Medicare Spending in 2022 | $4.6 billion | $974 million | $144 million |
| Average Spend per Claim in 2022 | $1,356.90 | $1,420.41 | $ 1,189.44 |

Sources: CRS Analysis of Centers for Medicare & Medicaid Services Medicare Part D Spending by Drug 2022; FDA.

Note: This table represents a subset of GLP-1 drugs available under Medicare Part D to provide a snapshot of Part D utilization. This table shows the most recent publicly available data.

## Coverage Under Enhanced Alternative Plans

Part D sponsors also may offer enhanced alternative (EA) Part D plans in addition to their basic plans. CMS defines an EA plan as coverage that includes the standard prescription coverage as well as supplemental benefits.

Approximately 75% of Medicare Part D beneficiaries are enrolled in EA plans. Some EA plans offer a lower deductible and/or reduced enrollee cost sharing. Another example of a qualifying supplemental benefit is coverage of drugs that are excluded from the definition of a Part D drug, such as a GLP-1 drugs approved by the FDA for weight loss but not for T2DM or CVD. An EA plan also could potentially allow a beneficiary to access a GLP-1 drug that is currently covered by Part D for off-label use, such as weight loss. There is no requirement that EA plans offer GLP-1 drugs, and beneficiaries who choose an EA plan may be required to pay a higher monthly premium in order to access its broader formulary.

## Barriers to Access

If a Part D plan covers a GLP-1 drug, either under the standard benefit for T2DM and/or CVD or under an enhanced plan for weight loss, enrollees still may experience varying levels of cost sharing or formulary restrictions. Plans can place drugs on different tiers within their formularies, with higher tiers associated with greater enrollee cost sharing. If beneficiaries are facing difficulties accessing a GLP-1 drug, they can apply for exceptions to gain access to a drug not on their plan's formulary or lower their cost sharing if the drug is on a high tier.

Plans also can use drug utilization management strategies, such as step therapy and prior authorization, that would require patients to go through additional processes before being prescribed a GLP-1 drug. Both Blue Cross Blue Shield and UnitedHealthCare now require prior authorization for GLP-1 drug coverage under their MA products, to ensure only individuals with a diagnosis of T2DM are using these drugs. Despite these restrictions, there are still widespread shortages for many GLP-1 medications, with even individuals who have T2DM struggling to access them.

## Congressional Policy Considerations

As the use of GLP-1 drugs expands beyond diabetes management to cardiovascular and obesity treatment, the associated costs and coverage policies likely will continue to be a focal point facing policymakers. Congressional actions in the coming years could significantly shape the future landscape of Medicare coverage for GLP-1 drugs, with potential implications for both the future cost of the program and the health outcomes of beneficiaries.

Under the current design of the Medicare Part D benefit, many beneficiaries do not have access to GLP-1 drugs for the treatment of obesity, unless they have another qualifying condition such as T2DM or CVD. In the 118th Congress, some have expressed interest in expanding the permitted utilization of these drugs under Medicare Part D.

H.R. 4818, the Treat and Reduce Obesity Act of 2023, would expand Medicare Part D coverage to include prescription drugs for the treatment of obesity. Under this bill, individuals who are not obese but are overweight and have certain comorbidities also would qualify for coverage of GLP-1 drugs. An amended H.R. 4818 was voted out of committee in June 2024. S. 2407, a companion bill, was introduced in the Senate in July 2023.

In addition to interest in expanding access to these drugs, there has been scrutiny on their cost. As shown in Table 1, Medicare expenditures on Ozempic alone exceeded $4 billion in 2022. Although these drugs are new, current studies suggest that patients have to continue using the drugs to sustain their weight loss. Goldman Sachs has forecast a $100 billion worldwide market for obesity drugs by 2030. The Inflation Reduction Act of 2022 (P.L. 117- 169) authorized the Secretary of the Department of Health and Human Services to negotiate prices for certain high- cost drugs. Although no GLP-1 drugs were selected in the first round of negotiations, these drugs' high costs and the prevalence of diabetes among Medicare beneficiaries make them possible candidates for future negotiations.

The financial impact of legislation related to GLP-1 drugs is difficult to predict. In October 2023, the Congressional Budget Office (CBO) issued a request for new research in the area of obesity. According to CBO, the budgetary effect of such legislation would depend on prices as well as any effect of usage on other health care spending: "In CBO's assessment, Medicare's coverage of anti-obesity medications at their current prices (accounting for rebates and discounts) would increase overall federal spending." CBO added that there is little information on longer-term effects of the drugs.

Chapter 21

# Financial Help for Diabetes Care*


## National Institute of Diabetes and Digestive and Kidney Diseases


Diabetes management is expensive. According to the American Diabetes Association (ADA), the average cost of health care for a person with diabetes is $16,752 a year—more than twice the cost of health care for a person without diabetes [1].

Many people who have diabetes need help paying for their care. You can find help through private or government health insurance, local programs, patient support groups, and medicine-assistance programs. You can also find ways to save money on diabetes medicines and supplies.

## What Health Insurance Plans Cover People with Diabetes?

Health insurance helps pay for medical care, including the cost of diabetes care. Your health insurance options are

- private health insurance, which includes group and individual health insurance
- government health insurance, such as Medicare External link, Medicaid External link, the Children's Health Insurance Program

* This is an edited, reformatted and augmented version of National Institute of Diabetes and Digestive and Kidney Diseases Publication.


In: Comprehensive Diabetes Care
Editor: Joseph S. Green
ISBN: 979-8-89530-772-4

External link (CHIP), TRICARE External link, and veterans' health care programs External link

Under current law, health insurance companies can't refuse to cover you or charge you more just because you have a "pre-existing condition External link"—that is, a health problem you had before the date that new health coverage starts.

Changes to insurance rules happen often and may affect your health insurance choices. Learn more or get help with your health insurance questions through

- HealthCare.gov External link , the federal marketplace, 1-800-318-2596, TTY: 1-855-889-4325
- the Center for Consumer Information & Insurance Oversight Program External link , which offers help by phone, by email, or at walk-in locations
- the state health insurance resources tool External link of the American Diabetes Association
- the National Association of Insurance Commissioners External link
- Learn key terms about diabetes costs, insurance, and financial aid.

## Compare Coverage for Diabetes Care

When choosing a health insurance plan, ask about every service and supply you'll need to manage your diabetes. Does the plan cover the medicines, supplies, and devices that you are using, and, if not, what are the alternatives? What does the plan pay? How much will you need to pay out of pocket? Consider

- each prescription medicine you need
- diabetes supplies and devices, such as an insulin pump
- diabetes lab tests and screening exams
- medical office visits, nutrition counseling, and specialists, such as eye doctors
- copayments and deductibles

- health care providers—do your providers participate in the plan, or will you have to change providers or pay more to see your current providers because they are out of network?

Ask for a Summary of Benefits and Coverage, which explains the plan in plain language, including free preventive services. This summary may include a coverage example for managing diabetes.

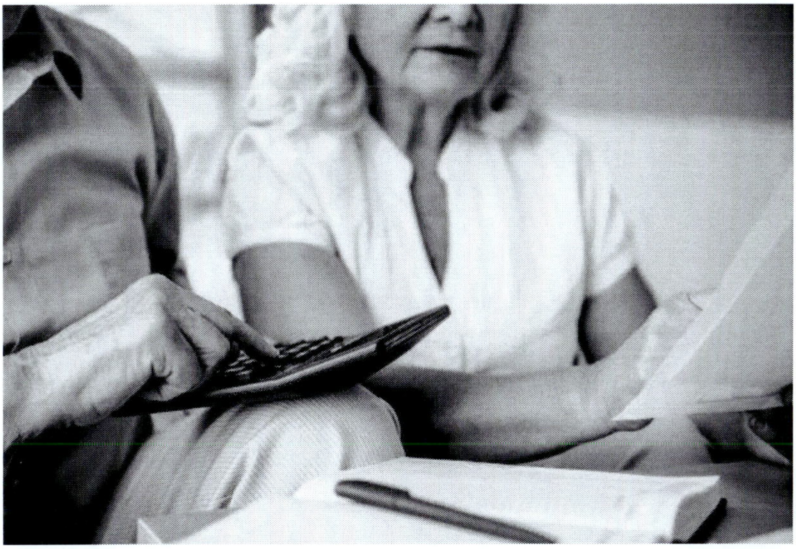

When looking for health insurance, determine if each plan pays for the services and supplies you need to manage your diabetes.

## Private Health Insurance

Insurance companies sell private health insurance plans. Two types of private health insurance are

- Group health insurance. People buy this kind of health insurance through their employer, union, or a family member's employer or union. Professional or alumni groups may also offer group health insurance, which may be helpful for people who are self-employed.

- Individual health insurance. People buy this coverage for themselves and their families.
- HealthCare.gov is one way to find, compare, and buy individual insurance plans in most states—or connect to your state's insurance marketplace. HealthCare.gov also
    - tells you whether you qualify for a premium tax credit External link that lowers your monthly premiums and cost-sharing reductions External link that lower your out-of-pocket costs. Only people who buy plans through HealthCare.gov or a state exchange can get premium tax credits or cost-sharing reductions.
    - lists the yearly open enrollment period when you can choose or change your plan
    - lists the life events that allow you to buy insurance any time of year
- Learn more about Healthcare.gov online External link or by calling 1-800-318-2596, TTY: 1-855-889-4325.
- Insurance companies, agents, brokers, and online insurance stores are other ways to find and buy individual health insurance plans. Learn how to find a trustworthy insurance company at USA.gov External link or by calling 1-844-USA-GOV1 (1-844-872-4681).

## Preventive Care

You may be eligible for some important preventative services External link at no additional cost to you. These services can help find and treat health problems early. For example, adults who are overweight or who have obesity or high blood pressure may be able to get diabetes screening tests at no out-of-pocket cost. Adults and children may be able to get obesity screening and weight-management counseling at no out-of-pocket cost.

## Keeping Health Insurance After Leaving a Job

A federal law called COBRA allows you to stay on your employer's health plan for 18 to 36 months after leaving a job. You'll pay both your own monthly premiums and the employer's portion, so your cost is likely to be higher than before.

- People with a disability may be able to extend COBRA coverage for an extra 11 months.
- COBRA may also cover young adults who "age out" of a parent's policy when they reach the age limit of 26.
- Learn more about COBRA online External link or call the U.S. Department of Labor at 1–866–4–USA–DOL (1–866–487–2365).

## Federal Government Health Insurance

### What is Medicare?

Medicare is a federal health insurance program that pays health care costs for eligible people who are

- age 65 or older
- under age 65 with certain disabilities
- of any age with end-stage renal disease—total and permanent kidney failure that requires a kidney transplant or blood-filtering treatments called dialysis External link

## What Health Plans Does Medicare Offer?

*Medicare* has four parts:

- Part A External link , or hospital insurance, covers hospital stays, skilled nursing homes, hospice care, and some home health care. Part A has no premium for those who have paid enough Medicare taxes. Part A has a deductible, which is an amount you pay for your care each year before the plan begins to pay.
- Part B External link, or medical insurance, covers doctor visits, outpatient care, some home health care, medical equipment including insulin pumps, and some preventive services. You pay a monthly premium based on your income. After you pay the deductible each year, Part B pays 80 percent for most covered services, and you pay 20 percent.

  - Part B covers the Medicare Diabetes Prevention Program External link (MDPP) for members with prediabetes. The MDPP provides healthy eating and physical activity training sessions and support over 12 months, which research shows can sharply lower diabetes risk.
- *Medicare Advantage Plans External link* are private insurance plans that combine Medicare Part A and B benefits with extras such as medicine coverage. The Federal Government sets the basic rules for Medicare Advantage plans. However, you'll find many options for extra services, along with different premiums and copayments. Covered services External link can change from year to year. Ask about
  - whether you need a referral to see a specialist
  - whether you must use doctors, clinics, or suppliers that belong to one plan, also called "in network" providers
- *Part D External link*, or prescription drug coverage, is optional coverage offered by private companies, with approval from Medicare. Your premiums, deductible, additional costs, and covered medicines depend on which Part D plan you choose. You may qualify for lower Part D premiums and lower medicine costs, depending on your income and resources. Learn more about the Medicare Extra Help Program online External link.

Other Medicare health plans are available with special rules or for specific groups of people. Medicare offers more information online External link. These alternate health plans include

- *Medicare Cost Plans,* which often include payments for out-of-network providers
- *Medicare Demonstrations and Pilot Projects,* which test improvements in Medicare coverage and care
- *Programs of All-Inclusive Care for the Elderly (PACE*), which combine medical, social, and long-term care services for frail people who live in the community
- *Medication Therapy Management Programs*, which can help you learn how to manage your medications if you're in a Medicare drug plan

Learn more about benefits, rules, and coverage details at Medicare.gov External link or by calling 1-800-MEDICARE (1-800-633-4227).

## Which Diabetes Services and Supplies Does Medicare Cover?

Medicare Part B and Part D cover many diabetes services and supplies. You may first need to pay a deductible, copayment, or coinsurance. Some services are free if your doctor orders them.

Medicare Part B helps pay for

- diabetes screening tests for people at risk of developing diabetes
- diabetes self-management training External link
- diabetes supplies such as glucose monitors, test strips, and lancets
- certain continuous glucose monitors and supplies
- counseling to help people who have obesity lose weight
- eye exams to check for glaucoma and diabetic retinopathy
- flu and pneumonia shots
- foot exams and treatment for people with diabetes
- insulin pumps and insulin that will be used with an insulin pump
- medical nutrition therapy services for people with diabetes or kidney disease
- therapeutic shoes or inserts

Medicare Part D helps pay for

- diabetes medications
- diabetes supplies such as needles and syringes for injecting insulin
- insulin, except for insulin used with an insulin pump, which is covered by Medicare Part B

Check your own plan to learn exactly what is covered. Each plan, especially Medicare Advantage Plans, may offer different coverage for diabetes care. Read more about Medicare's diabetes coverage rules External link (PDF, 671 KB) online or call 1-800-MEDICARE (1-800-633-4227).

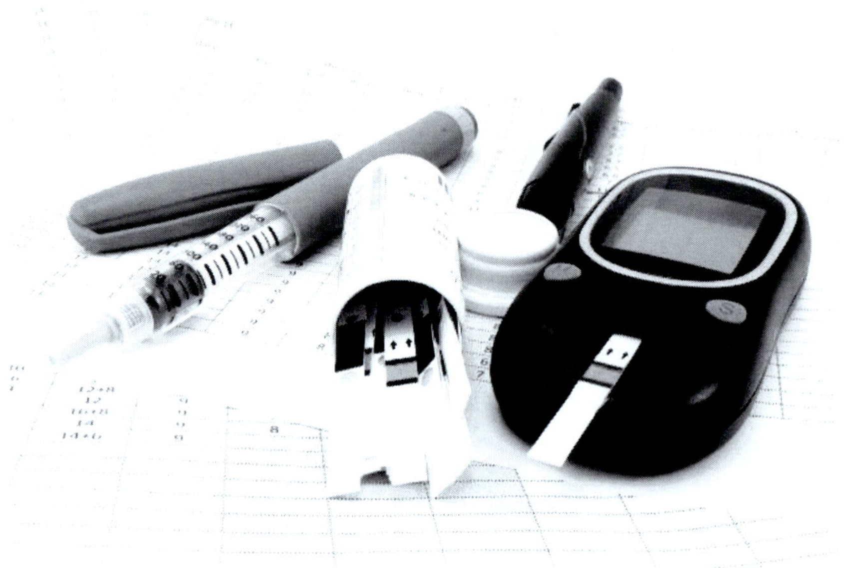

Medicare pays for many diabetes supplies and drugs under Part B and Part D, which is the optional, extra coverage for medicines.

## What Is Medigap?

Medigap plans help pay costs that are not covered by Medicare, such as deductibles, copayments, and coinsurance. You can buy a Medigap policy from a licensed insurance company in your home state. Learn more online about Medigap rules, benefits, deadlines, and premiums External link.

## What Other Federal Programs Can Help?

The following federal programs can provide more resources for people with diabetes

- U.S. Department of Veterans Affairs External link
- TRICARE External link
- Indian Health Service External link

- Hill-Burton Free and Reduced-cost Health Care Program External link
- Bureau of Primary Health Care External link
- Social Security Administration
- Social Security Disability Insurance (SSDI)
- Supplemental Security Income (SSI)
- Women, Infants, and Children (WIC)

The Social Security Administration can provide financial help through two programs

- SSDI pays a monthly amount to people who can't work and have paid enough Social Security taxes. If an illness or injury keeps you out of work for at least a year, SSDI payments may be an option.
- SSI pays a monthly amount to disabled children and adults who earn little and don't have many financial assets. A person who gets SSI may be able to get Medicaid and food stamps External link through the Supplemental Nutrition Assistance Program (SNAP), too.

Read more about both SSDI and SSI and how to apply at ssa.gov External link or by calling 1–800–772–1213, TTY: 1–800–325–0778.

*WIC* serves mothers and children who are at risk for poor nutrition or hunger. This includes low-income women who are pregnant, breastfeeding, or recently had a baby, as well as infants and children up to age 5. Pregnant women who have gestational diabetes may qualify for help through the WIC program. WIC provides

- supplemental foods
- health care referrals
- nutrition education
- breastfeeding information

Learn more about WIC online External link, or call the WIC's headquarters at 703-305-2062.

## State Government Health Insurance

### What is Medicaid?

Medicaid is a health insurance program funded by the Federal Government and state governments for people with low incomes and few assets. Each state runs its own program based on federal rules. Some states cover more services than federal rules require. Many states expanded Medicaid in recent years to cover more people, including low-income adults without dependent children.

Find out whether you qualify for Medicaid in your state, or apply for coverage through

- HealthCare.gov External link, 1-800-318-2596, TTY: 1-855-889-4325
- National Association of Medicaid Directors state agency locator External link

Learn more at Medicaid.gov External link or call 1-877-267-2323 (TTY: 1-866-226-1819).

### What Is the Children's Health Insurance Program (CHIP)?

CHIP offers free or low-cost Medicaid to children whose parents earn too much for Medicaid but not enough to pay for a private health plan. In some states, CHIP may also cover pregnant women and parents. Learn whether your family members qualify for CHIP through HealthCare.gov External link or your state's Medicaid or CHIP agency External link.

Learn more about CHIP at www.insurekidsnow.gov External link or call 1–877–543–7669.

### What Other State Programs Can Help?

Medicare Savings Programs in certain states may pay Medicare premiums, deductibles, and coinsurance if a person has a low income and few assets. Learn more online External link.

State Health Insurance Assistance Programs (SHIPs) give advice about health insurance in every state to people who have Medicare. SHIP counselors can help you choose the best plan for your needs. Find a SHIP counselor at ShiptaCenter.org External link or call 1-877-839-2675.

State Pharmaceutical Assistance Programs help pay for prescription medicines in certain states. Learn what programs are available in your state. External link

## Local Resources for Care and Costs

Local health departments and clinics can help people with diabetes find medical care at little or no cost. Search for help near you at FindaHealthCenter.hrsa.gov External link, or call 1-877-464-4772; TTY: 1-877-897-991.

Charitable groups in your community may offer financial help for diabetes care

- Lions Clubs International can help with vision care: LionsClubs.org External link
- Shriners Hospitals offer free treatment for children: ShrinersHospitalsforChildren.org External link
- Kiwanis clubs run service projects to help children and communities: Kiwanis.org External link

## Help Paying for Diabetes Medicines and Supplies

Don't hesitate to speak up and talk with your health care team if you have trouble paying for your diabetes medicines and supplies. Ask if there are generic versions of the medicines you need for managing diabetes, blood pressure, and cholesterol. Generic medicines are cheaper than brand-name medicines.

Even when generic versions of medicines aren't available, there may be different, less expensive medicines available to treat diabetes, blood pressure, and cholesterol. If you can't afford a medicine, ask your team if you can switch to a different, less expensive medicine.

Your team may suggest other ways to help you save money, such as using free samples of glucose test strips or other supplies or contacting local programs that may provide financial support.

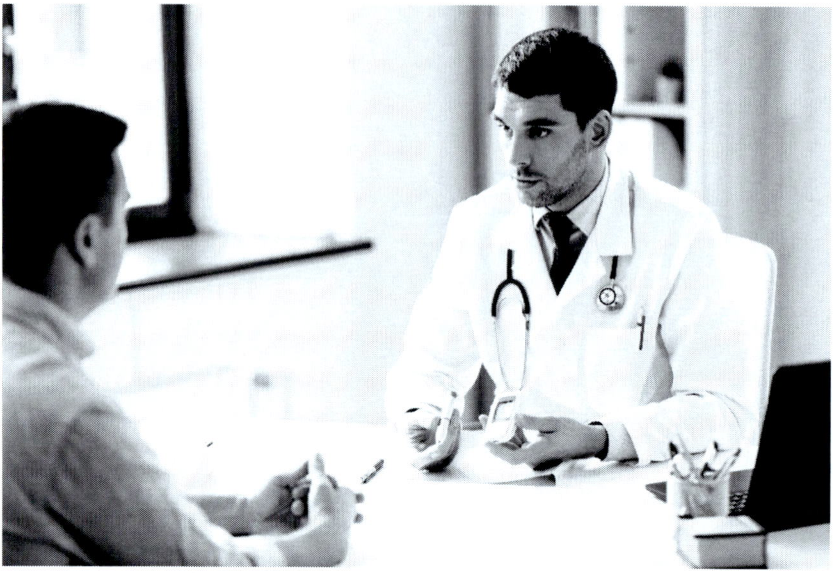

Talk with your health care team if you have trouble paying for your diabetes medicines and supplies.

Drug discount programs may help you find the medicines you need for free or a lower cost. Try these resources

- BenefitsCheckUp.org External link. Seniors with limited incomes can search for help with medicines, health care, rent, and other needs through this service of the National Council on Aging.
- NeedyMeds.org External link. This organization lists programs that help pay for medicines and supplies. You can search by medicine or manufacturer name.
- Partnership for Prescription Assistance (PPARX.org External link). People who don't have insurance coverage for prescriptions may find their medicines and supplies for free or at low cost through PPARX.org.
- RxAssist.org External link lists drug-company assistance programs, state programs, discount drug cards, copay help, and more.

- Rx Outreach is a nonprofit, mail-order pharmacy that provides affordable medicine to people in need through its website, RxOutreach.org External link , or by phone at 1-888-RX0-1234 (1-888-796-1234).

Websites can make it easier to find the exact medicine or supply you need at the lowest cost. Look for reputable websites that sell the same high-quality medicines as your local pharmacy.

Providers strongly advise against skipping doses of medicine or leaving some prescriptions unfilled to save money.

## Help Paying for Prosthetic Care

People who have had an amputation may get help paying for rehabilitation and a prosthesis.

Organizations that may help include

- Amputee Coalition External link
  Phone: 1-888-AMP-KNOW (1-888-267-5669)
- Limbs for Life Foundation External link

Phone: 1-888-235-5462 or 405-843-5171

## Help Paying for Kidney Dialysis and Transplantation

Kidney failure may be a complication of diabetes. People of any age with kidney failure can get Medicare if they meet certain criteria. Learn more about Financial Help for Treatment of Kidney Failure.

## Help for College Students with Diabetes

College students who have diabetes-related disabilities may face both the costs of tuition and medical expenses. These expenses may include special equipment and health costs not covered by insurance. Special equipment and support services may be available at your college, through community organizations, your state vocational rehabilitation agency, or specific disability organizations.

The HEATH Resource Center External link offers information about financial aid and other types of support for college students with disabilities.

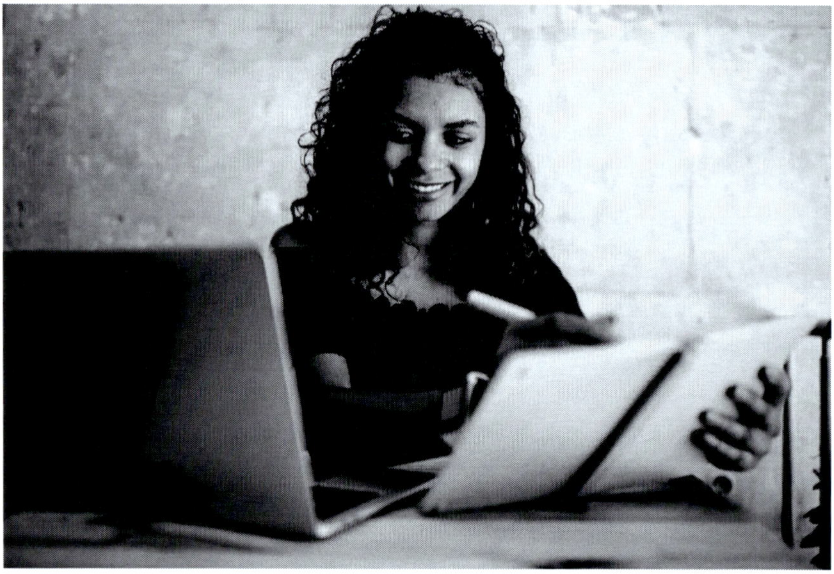

College students with diabetes may qualify for financial help with tuition and medical expenses.

## Assistive Technology for Living with Diabetes

Assistive technology is any device that assists or helps someone with a disability function more safely, effectively, and independently at home, at work, and in the community. Assistive technology may include

- computers with features that let people with disabilities use them more easily
- low-vision devices, such as magnifiers
- adaptive equipment, such as wheelchairs
- bathroom changes, such as adding grab bars or shower seats

The following organizations offer information, awareness, resources, and training in assistive technology

- Able Data
  Phone: 1-800-227-0216; TTY: 703-992-8313
- United Cerebral Palsy External link
- Phone: 1-800-872-5827 or 202-776-0406

## Key Terms

Some terms listed here have many meanings; only those meanings that relate to the financial and medical aspects of diabetes and its management and treatment are included.

*coinsurance:* an amount a person may still need to pay after a deductible for health care. The amount is most often a percentage, such as 20 percent.

*copay (or copayment):* an amount a person may have to pay for health care. A copay is often a set fee. A person might pay $10 or $20 for a health care provider's visit or prescription.

*deductible:* an amount a person must pay for health care or prescriptions before the health plan(s) will pay.

*network:* a group of health care providers that gives members a discount. Some plans pay for health care and prescriptions only if received from a network provider.

*out of network:* health care providers who are not in a plan's network. In some health plans, health care and prescriptions cost more if received from these providers.

*pre-existing condition:* a health problem a person had before the date that new health coverage starts.

*premium:* an amount a person must pay periodically—monthly or quarterly—for Medicare, other health plan, or drug plan coverage.

## Reference

[1] American Diabetes Association. Economic costs of diabetes in the U.S. in 2017 *NIH external link*. *Diabetes Care.* 2018;41(5):917–928.

Chapter 22

# Your Glucose Meter*

## U.S. Food and Drug Administration

Meters come in different sizes. Meters also come with different features. Some meters let you track and print out your test results. Others have audio and larger screens to help people who have problems seeing. The meter you choose should fit your lifestyle and your needs.

Glucose meters test and record how much sugar (called glucose) is in your blood. They help you track your blood sugar level at different times of the day and night.

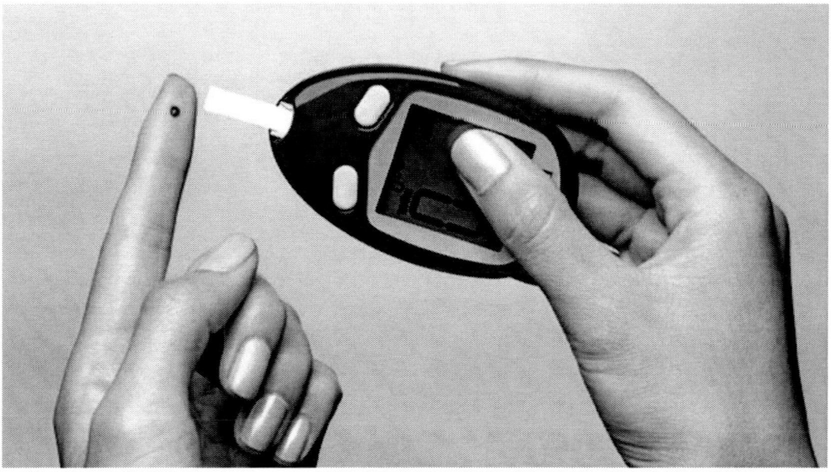

Meters can help you know how well your diabetes medicines are working.

---

* This is an edited, reformatted and augmented version of U.S. Food and Drug Administration Publication, dated 2018.

In: Comprehensive Diabetes Care
Editor: Joseph S. Green
ISBN: 979-8-89530-772-4

They can also help teach you how the food you eat and exercise can change your blood sugar level.

Three things you will need with your meter:

- Lancet — A small needle used to get a drop of blood from your finger or other part of your body.
- Test Strip — The strip goes in the meter. You put a drop of blood on the strip.
- Control Solution — Liquid used to make sure your meter is working right.

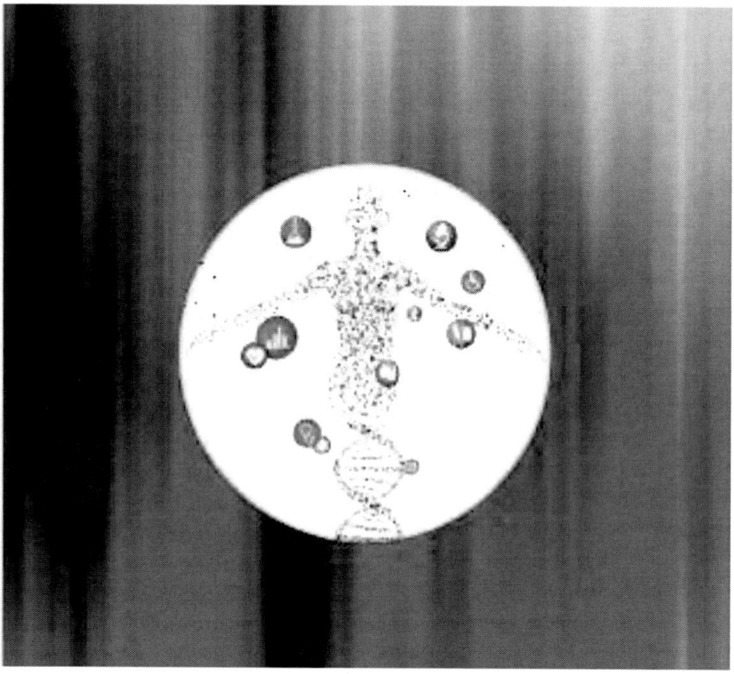

FDA Office of Women's Health; www.fda.gov/womensdiabetes

## 7 Helpful Tips for Testing Your Blood Sugar

1) Read the directions for your meter and test strips before you use them.
2) Wash your hands before you check your blood sugar. Food or juice on your fingers could make the meter give you the wrong result.

3) Use the right test strip for your meter. The meter may not work right or may give you the wrong result if you use the wrong test strip.
4) Write down your results and the date and time you tested. Do this even if your meter tracks your numbers. Take the results with you when you go to your doctor.
5) Clean your meter as directed. Some cleaning products may harm your meter.
6) Ask your healthcare provider if your medicines will change your blood sugar. If you are a kidney patient on dialysis, the dialysis solution can change your blood sugar.
7) Take your meter with you when you go to your doctor. This way you can test your blood sugar in front of the doctor or nurse to make sure you are doing it the right way. Your healthcare provider may be able to print out your blood sugar results from your meter.

This fact sheet was developed by the FDA Office of Women's Health.
To get other FDA diabetes resources, go to:
www.fda.gov/womensdiabetes

# Index

## L



## M



## N



## O



## P



## Q



## R

## W



## Y